T0264438

Food Animal Neurology

Editor

KEVIN E. WASHBURN

VETERINARY CLINICS
OF NORTH AMERICA:
FOOD ANIMAL PRACTICE

www.vetfood.theclinics.com

Consulting Editor
ROBERT A. SMITH

March 2017 • Volume 33 • Number 1

ELSEVIER

1600 John F. Kennedy Boulevard • Suite 1800 • Philadelphia, Pennsylvania, 19103-2899

http://www.vetfood.theclinics.com

VETERINARY CLINICS OF NORTH AMERICA: FOOD ANIMAL PRACTICE Volume 33, Number 1
March 2017 ISSN 0749-0720, ISBN-13: 978-0-323-50989-3

Editor: Katie Pfaff
Developmental Editor: Meredith Clinton

© **2017 Elsevier Inc. All rights reserved.**

This periodical and the individual contributions contained in it are protected under copyright by Elsevier, and the following terms and conditions apply to their use:

Photocopying
Single photocopies of single articles may be made for personal use as allowed by national copyright laws. Permission of the Publisher and payment of a fee is required for all other photocopying, including multiple or systematic copying, copying for advertising or promotional purposes, resale, and all forms of document delivery. Special rates are available for educational institutions that wish to make photocopies for non-profit educational classroom use. For information on how to seek permission visit www.elsevier.com/permissions or call: (+44) 1865 843830 (UK)/(+1) 215 239 3804 (USA).

Derivative Works
Subscribers may reproduce tables of contents or prepare lists of articles including abstracts for internal circulation within their institutions. Permission of the Publisher is required for resale or distribution outside the institution. Permission of the Publisher is required for all other derivative works, including compilations and translations (please consult www.elsevier.com/permissions).

Electronic Storage or Usage
Permission of the Publisher is required to store or use electronically any material contained in this periodical, including any article or part of an article (please consult www.elsevier.com/permissions). Except as outlined above, no part of this publication may be reproduced, stored in a retrieval system or transmitted in any form or by any means, electronic, mechanical, photocopying, recording or otherwise, without prior written permission of the Publisher.

Notice
No responsibility is assumed by the Publisher for any injury and/or damage to persons or property as a matter of products liability, negligence or otherwise, or from any use or operation of any methods, products, instructions or ideas contained in the material herein. Because of rapid advances in the medical sciences, in particular, independent verification of diagnoses and drug dosages should be made.

Although all advertising material is expected to conform to ethical (medical) standards, inclusion in this publication does not constitute a guarantee or endorsement of the quality or value of such product or of the claims made of it by its manufacturer.

Veterinary Clinics of North America: Food Animal Practice (ISSN 0749-0720) is published in March, July, and November by Elsevier Inc., 360 Park Avenue South, New York, NY 10010-1710. Subscription prices are $240.00 per year (domestic individuals), $386.00 per year (domestic institutions), $100.00 per year (domestic students/residents), $265.00 per year (Canadian individuals), $509.00 per year (Canadian institutions), $335.00 per year (international individuals), $509.00 per year (international institutions), and $165.00 per year (international and Canadian students/ residents). To receive student/resident rate, orders must be accompanied by name of affiliated institution, date of term, and the signature of program/residency coordinator on institution letterhead. *Clinics* subscription prices. All prices are subject to change without notice. **POSTMASTER:** Send address changes to *Veterinary Clinics of North America*: *Food Animal Practice*, Elsevier Health Sciences Division, Subscription Customer Service, 3251 Riverport Lane, Maryland Heights, MO 63043. Customer Service (orders, claims, online, change of address): Elsevier Health Sciences Division, Subscription **Customer Service, 3251 Riverport Lane, Maryland Heights, MO 63043. Tel: 1-800-654-2452 (U.S. and Canada); 314-447-8871 (ouside U.S. and Canada). Fax: 314-447-8029. E-mail: journalscustomerservice-usa@elsevier.com (for print support); journalsonlinesupport-usa@elsevier.com (for online support).**

Reprints. For copies of 100 or more, of articles in this publication, please contact the Commercial Reprints Department, Elsevier Inc., 360 Park Avenue South, New York, NY 10010-1710. Tel.: 212-633-3874; Fax: 212-633-3820; E-mail: reprints@elsevier.com.

Veterinary Clinics of North America: Food Animal Practice is covered in *Current Contents/Agriculture, Biology and Environmental Sciences, MEDLINE/PubMed (Index Medicus), and Excerpta Medica.*

Contributors

CONSULTING EDITOR

ROBERT A. SMITH, DVM, MS
Diplomate, American Board of Veterinary Practitioners; Veterinary Research and Consulting Services, LLC, Greeley, Colorado

EDITOR

KEVIN E. WASHBURN, DVM
Diplomate, American College of Veterinary Internal Medicine (Large Animal Internal Medicine); Diplomate, American Board of Veterinary Practitioners (Food Animal Practice); Professor, Department of Large Animal Clinical Sciences, Food Animal Medicine, Texas A&M University, College of Veterinary Medicine and Biomedical Sciences, College Station, Texas

AUTHORS

MÉLANIE J. BOILEAU, DVM, MS
Associate Professor, Food Animal Medicine and Surgery, Veterinary Clinical Sciences, College of Veterinary Medicine, Oklahoma State University, Stillwater, Oklahoma

VINCENT DORE, DMV, MS
Department of Population Health and Pathobiology, College of Veterinary Medicine, North Carolina State University, Raleigh, North Carolina

GILLES FECTEAU
Diplomate, American College of Veterinary Internal Medicine; Full Professor, Université de Montréal, Saint-Hyacinthe, Québec, Canada

LISLE W. GEORGE, DVM, PhD
Diplomate, American College of Veterinary Internal Medicine; Professor Emeritus, University of California Davis, School of Veterinary Medicine, Davis, California

PHILIPPA GIBBONS, BVetMed(Hons), MS, MRCVS
Diplomate, American College of Veterinary Internal Medicine (Large Animal); Clinical Assistant Professor, Food Animal Medicine, Large Animal Clinical Sciences, Texas A&M University, College of Veterinary Medicine and Biomedical Sciences, College Station, Texas

JOHN GILLIAM, DVM, MS
Clinical Associate Professor of Food Animal Production Medicine and Field Services, Veterinary Clinical Sciences, College of Veterinary Medicine, Oklahoma State University, Stillwater, Oklahoma

AMANDA K. HARTNACK, DVM, MS, BA
Assistant Professor, Food Animal Surgery, Department of Large Animal Clinical Sciences, Texas A&M University, College Station, Texas

JOHN R. MIDDLETON, DVM, PhD
Diplomate, American College of Veterinary Internal Medicine; Professor, Department of Veterinary Medicine and Surgery, College of Veterinary Medicine, University of Missouri, Columbia, Missouri

DUSTY W. NAGY, DVM, MS, PhD
Diplomate, American College of Veterinary Internal Medicine; Associate Teaching Professor, College of Veterinary Medicine, University of Missouri, Columbia, Missouri

GENE A. NILES, DVM, MS
Diplomate, American Board of Veterinary Toxicology; Director, Rocky Ford Branch, Veterinary Diagnostic Laboratory System, Colorado State University, Rocky Ford, Colorado

JOANE PARENT, DMV, MVetSc
Diplomate, American College of Veterinary Internal Medicine (Neurology); Full Professor, Université de Montréal, Saint-Hyacinthe, Québec, Canada

GEOF SMITH, DVM, MS, PhD
Diplomate, American College of Veterinary Internal Medicine; Professor of Ruminant Medicine, Department of Population Health and Pathobiology, College of Veterinary Medicine, North Carolina State University, Raleigh, North Carolina

KEVIN E. WASHBURN, DVM
Diplomate, American College of Veterinary Internal Medicine (Large Animal Internal Medicine); Diplomate, American Board of Veterinary Practitioners (Food Animal Practice); Professor, Department of Large Animal Clinical Sciences, Food Animal Medicine, Texas A&M University, College of Veterinary Medicine and Biomedical Sciences, College Station, Texas

Contents

In this article, the neurologic examination of ruminants is reviewed. The proposed approach is simple, although thorough and methodical. The bovine veterinary practitioner should be able to efficiently assess the nervous system to rule out a primary neurologic disorder. Simple observations and procedures are suggested to allow evaluation of the nervous system. The appropriate method and interpretation are reviewed as well as the danger of misinterpretation.

A variety of diagnostic tests can be used to help further characterize and diagnose neurologic disease in ruminant species. Cerebrospinal fluid is easily collected, and analysis can help in defining the broad category of disease. Diagnostic imaging, including radiography, myelography, ultrasonography, computed tomography, and MRI, have all been used to varying degrees in ruminants. Advanced cross-sectional imaging techniques have the capacity to aid greatly in diagnosis, but their cost can often be prohibitive. Currently, electrodiagnostic tests are not well evaluated or used in the diagnosis of neurologic disease in ruminants.

As stated many times throughout this issue, localization of the origin of neurologic deficits in ruminants is paramount to successful diagnosis and prognosis. This article serves as a guide to answer 2 questions that should be asked when presented with a ruminant with neurologic dysfunction: is the lesion rostral or caudal to the foramen magnum, and does the animal have primary neurologic disease? The answers to these 2 broad questions begin the thought processes to more specifically describe the location and nature of the dysfunction. Challenges often facing the diagnostician include economic constraints, size of the animal, and unruly behavior.

Video content accompanies this article at http://www.vetfood.
theclinics.com.

Neurologic diseases of the cerebrum are relatively common in cattle. In calves, the primary cerebral disorders are polioencephalomalacia, meningitis, and sodium toxicity. Because diagnostic testing is not always readily available, the practitioner must often decide on a course of treatment based on knowledge of the likely disease, as well as his or her own clinical experience. This is particularly true with neurologic diseases in which the prognosis is often poor and euthanasia may be the most humane outcome. This article reviews the most common diseases affecting the cerebrum of calves with a focus on pathophysiology, diagnosis, and treatment.

Although clinical impression suggests that cerebral disorders of adult ruminants are not very common, an understanding of the common differential diagnoses is important to maintaining animal and human health. The most common causes of cerebral dysfunction are metabolic, toxic, or infectious. Many of the diseases and disorders cannot be easily differentiated based on clinical signs or antemortem diagnostic tests alone. Knowing which diseases can be easily ruled in or out, and how, will help the practitioner make case management decisions and have broader impact through recognizing index cases of emergent diseases and reducing exposure to zoonotic pathogens.

Cerebellar disease can be congenital or acquired. Clinical signs of cerebellar disease include hypermetric gait in all limbs, normal to increased muscle tone, wide-based stance, swaying, intention tremor, and convulsions. Vestibular signs may be observed. Differential diagnoses for etiology include congenital (hypoplasia, abiotrophy, and lysosomal storage diseases), viral, bacterial, and toxic plants. Animals may present aborted as fetuses or stillborn, be affected at birth, develop disease at a few months old, or acquire the disease later in life.

Asymmetrical signs of brainstem disease occur relatively infrequently in ruminants. The most common differential diagnoses include listeriosis, otitis media/interna, and pituitary abscess syndrome. Although these conditions produce signs of brainstem dysfunction, the diseases can usually be differentiated based on historical findings and subtle clinical differences. Basic laboratory diagnostic tests are often not specific in the definitive diagnosis but may be supportive. Advanced imaging techniques have proven to be useful in the diagnosis of otitis media/interna. Presumptive clinical diagnosis is confirmed at necropsy. Treatment involves a prolonged course of antibiotic therapy but is unrewarding in cases of pituitary abscess syndrome.

In food animals, spinal cord damage is most commonly associated with infection or trauma. Antemortem diagnosis is based on clinical signs, history, cerebrospinal fluid analysis, and imaging. As clinical signs are often severe, and prognosis is grave, necropsy may provide a postmortem diagnosis. Peripheral nerve abnormalities are most often the result of trauma. Calving paralysis or paresis is the most common condition affecting the sciatic or obturator nerve and often concurrently involves the peroneal branch of the sciatic. Damage to peripheral nerves is often transient and resolves within a few days as long as the nerve is not severed.

This article discusses the etiology, mechanism of action, clinical signs, and diagnostic tests used to identify toxic agents that affect the nervous system of ruminants. The article is not intended to be an exhaustive review of each agent, but a reference for establishing a differential diagnosis when toxic agents are suspected as the cause of central nervous system disease in ruminants. The initial focus of the article is on agents that cause brain lesions consistent with polioencephalomalacia. Other neurotoxic disease agents include bovine bonkers, urea, organophosphate, organochlorine, cyanobacteria, zinc, aluminum, phosphide, metaldehyde, strychnine, botulism, tetanus, clostridium perfringens, and poisonous plants.

VETERINARY CLINICS OF NORTH AMERICA: FOOD ANIMAL PRACTICE

THE CLINICS ARE NOW AVAILABLE ONLINE!
Access your subscription at:
www.theclinics.com

Preface

A Practitioners Guide to Diseases and Conditions Leading to Neurologic Dysfunction in the Ruminant

 CrossMark

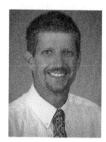

Kevin E. Washburn, DVM
Editor

Neurologic signs are often a challenge in our food and fiber animals due to multiple factors. The size and unruly behavior of some of these animals may hinder the performance of a full neurologic examination as well as the ability to practically perform ancillary diagnostic testing. These obstacles may lead to the inability of the diagnostician to achieve a definitive ante-mortem diagnosis. In addition, to add to the anxiety level of these cases, owners are often alarmed at the severity of the symptoms and know something is terribly wrong. Nevertheless, despite this seemingly discouraging and often frustrating scenario, as veterinary clinicians, our charge is to determine whether the signs are of primary (neoplasia) or secondary (metabolic, infectious, toxic, traumatic) in origin in order to address herd ramifications, animal welfare, and zoonotic potential. The determination of origin begins with a thorough history and localization of the lesion(s) by means of a neurologic examination. This regimen should narrow the differential list and determine the course of further diagnostic testing. If it is not physically or economically practical to pursue further diagnostic testing, by this point the diagnostician may well have enough information to achieve a solid working diagnosis. At the least, a working diagnosis allows the clinician to speak to prognosis and potential therapeutic intervention. However, in some scenarios, the diagnostician is left to "treat the treatable" based on the working diagnosis.

These articles are laid out by components of the nervous system from head to tail so that various conditions affecting that portion are addressed within. It is hoped that this systematic scheme will serve as a good reference once one has localized the lesion to aid the practitioner in ante-mortem diagnoses. These articles were written by ACVIM-boarded food and fiber animal clinicians in addition to one boarded toxicologist. I want

Vet Clin Food Anim 33 (2017) ix–x
http://dx.doi.org/10.1016/j.cvfa.2016.09.010
0749-0720/17/© 2016 Published by Elsevier Inc.

to thank them for their contributions and hope you find this issue to be a valuable resource. Although not much has changed in the understanding of the diseases and conditions described in this issue since the last issue in 2004, it is hoped that the manner in which it is presented will give the clinician a useful tool when one is confronted with neurologic dysfunction in food and fiber animals.

Kevin E. Washburn, DVM
Department of Large Animal Clinical Sciences
Texas A&M University
College of Veterinary Medicine and Biomedical Sciences
MS 4475, College Station
TX 77843-4475, USA

E-mail address:
kwashburn@cvm.tamu.edu

Neurologic Examination of the Ruminant

Gilles Fecteau[a],*, Joane Parent, DMV, MVetSc, ACVIM Neurology[a],
Lisle W. George, DVM, PhD[b]

KEYWORDS

- Bovine - Neurologic examination - Cattle - Ancillary tests - Ruminants

KEY POINTS

- The neurologic examination in the ruminant is part of a complete physical examination.
- With a few simple observations and clinical procedures, one should be able to rapidly evaluate the nervous system.
- A methodical approach allows for an efficient and thorough assessment of the nervous system.

INTRODUCTION

A detailed neurologic examination should be performed whenever the history, complaint, or physical finding suggests involvement of the nervous system.[1,2] The primary objective of the neurologic examination is to determine the area of the nervous system that is most likely affected. Precise description of the clinical signs is more important than trying to fit the observations to a specific disease. A methodical approach should be used to ensure that all nerves and reflexes are evaluated. The observations should be recorded in sufficient detail. As the condition evolves and the neurologic examination is repeated over time, the clinician can assess if there is improvement or deterioration. One cannot overemphasize the power of observation in food animal neurology. A thorough history is extremely important. Be aware that owners may omit relevant details on history or patient management.

Sensorium, gait and posture, placement spinal reflexes, pain perception, and cranial nerves (CNs) should be included in the neurologic examination. The neurological examination can be divided into specific steps/observations: (1) the mental status and (2) cranial nerves involving mainly the head (3) the gait and posture (4) the postural reactions (5) the spinal reflexes and (6) the response to pain.

Disclosure Statement: The authors have nothing to disclose.
[a] Département de Sciences Cliniques, Université de Montréal, 3200 Sicotte, Saint-Hyacinthe, Québec J2S 7C6, Canada; [b] University of California Davis, School of Veterinary Medicine, 425 Heron Pl, Davis, CA 95616, USA
* Corresponding author.
E-mail address: gilles.fecteau@umontreal.ca

0749-0720/17/© 2016 Elsevier Inc. All rights reserved.
vetfood.theclinics.com

STEP 1: MENTAL STATUS

The mental status evaluation provides the most important evidence in differentiating intracranial from extracranial lesion. Abnormalities of the brainstem or of the thalamo-cortex alter patients' behavior and interaction with the environment. Awareness of the examiner's presence and social interaction with herd mates are some key elements for examination of the mental status.

Brainstem: Arousal

This area is responsible for the animal's arousal. Changes resulting from brainstem disorders include stupor, somnolence, and coma, with deficits in cranial functions. The animal appears sedated. Although the animal is quieter than expected, it remains fully aware of its surroundings. This awareness also means that it will be responding as expected to environmental stimuli. Somnolence, however, can easily go unnoticed. It is important for the clinician to observe the animal arousal during history taking whenever there are CN deficits. There are 2 steps in the assessment of the mental status: first, before any stimulation and at distance from the animal and then when contact and stimulation are initiated. The final result of this examination is combined with the CN evaluation.

Thalamocortex: Behavior

The thalamocortex is responsible for cognitive function. Animals with lesions of the thalamus and cerebral cortex separate from the herd and fail to react to environmental stimuli. Other signs of thalamic or cortical disorders include head pressing, compulsive walking, head tilt, circling, and blindness. Animals with pituitary or suprahypophyseal lesions may have bradycardia.

Evaluate the thalamocortex by observing the patients' mental status, the menace response, nasal septum tactile responses, and stimulation and proprioceptive positioning. With severe cortical involvement, there is unawareness (the animal cannot be stimulated), cortical blindness (the pupillary reflexes are normal in the absence of menace responses), absent response to nasal septum stimulation, and proprioceptive deficits if they can be evaluated.

The mental status assessment was described earlier. The menace responses and proprioceptive positioning are described later. The nasal septum stimulation (Cranial Nerve V, thalamocortex) is described herein.

The nasal septum is the most sensitive region of the animal's head. When stimulating the nasal septum the animal may or may not blink, but the head is pulled away as a pain response. This stimulation should be done gently using cotton swabs or the small finger so as to reveal subtle differences between sides. Start with a gentle stimulus and gradually increase the strength of the stimulus going from side to side, until a consistent response (normal or not) is obtained. The nasal septum is the only area that consistently elicits a cortical response in the domestic species. It is best not to restrain the animal's head.

STEP 2: CRANIAL NERVES

Steps 1 and 2 are often performed in parallel. There are 12 pairs of CNs numbered I to XII, from the most rostral to the most caudal. Remembering the location of the nucleus for each CN helps localize the lesion when a centrally mediated CN deficit is observed.

Thalamocortex	I: Olfactory nerve
	II: Optic nerve
Midbrain	III: Oculomotor nerve
	IV: Trochlear nerve
Pons	V: Trigeminal motor nerve
Rostral medulla	V: Trigeminal sensory nerve
	VI: Abducent nerve
	VII: Facial nerve
	VIII: Vestibulo-cochlear nerve
Caudal Medulla	IX: Glossopharyngeal nerve
	X: Vagal nerve
	XI: Accessory nerve
	XII: Hypoglossal nerve

There are several methodical approaches to CN evaluation. The approach described later is based on a few simple procedures and observations. It provides rapid assessment, especially if the CNs are normal. All CNs are evaluated, with the exception of CNs I and XI, which cannot be adequately examined. Mentally counting from 1 to 12 ensures that each of the nerves has been evaluated.

Menace Response (Cranial Nerve II, Cortex, Cerebellum, Cranial Nerve VII)

The menace gesture must be performed 30 to 50 cm away from the animal's head. Air currents generated by the motion could stimulate touch perception on the eyelids, leading to a misinterpretation of the test. Compare the responses from each side. In the cow, there is no need to cover the eye that is not being examined, because the eyeballs are positioned laterally.

The menace responses evaluate not only the optic nerves but also the visual pathways in their entirety (retinas, optic nerves, optic chiasm, optic tracts, optic radiations, occipital cortices). It also requires intact cerebellum and CN VII. This response is not a reflex because it requires cerebral integration. The menace response is not innate and should be present by the end of the first week of life in farm animals.

Pupillary Light Reflexes (Cranial Nerve II, Cranial Nerve III)

Before the evaluation of the pupillary light reflexes, the pupils are examined for symmetry. Then, the reflexes are elicited. A strong light source must be used to stimulate pupillary constriction in normal animals. In order to perform the test, direct the light beam in a naso-temporal direction toward the maximum density of rods and cones. In the normal bovine, the pupils should constrict down to 3 to 5 mm. The retinas, optic nerves, and optic chiasm represent the afferent pathways of the pupillary light reflexes, whereas the oculomotor nerves (CN III) are the efferent pathways.

Position of the Eye in the Orbit and Eye Movement (Cranial Nerve III, IV, and VI) and Physiologic Nystagmus (Cranial Nerves III, IV, and VI, Medial Longitudinal Fasciculus, Cranial Nerve VIII)

Observe the eyes with the head erect and stationary. Note any nystagmus or strabismus. Nerves III, IV, and VI are evaluated as a functional unit. Presence of a strabismus indicates a nerve deficit. With CN VIII, the 3 nerves are also responsible for conjugate eye movements. Eliciting the physiologic nystagmus evaluates eye movement. In order to examine the conjugate eye movements, face the animal while moving the head horizontally. The eyes will have a nystagmus with the quick phase directed toward the head movement. Physiologic nystagmus will cease immediately after the head positioning changes have stopped. Abnormal nystagmus will continue while the patients' head is still.

Palpebral Reflexes (Cranial Nerve V, Cranial Nerve VII) and Symmetry of the Face (Cranial Nerve VII)

In these reflexes, CN V is the afferent limb (sensory), whereas CN VII is the efferent limb (motor). Examine the ears, eyelids, lip commissures, and nostrils for symmetry and function. Assess the ophthalmic branch of the trigeminal nerve by touching the medial canthus and observing a reflexive eyelid closure. Assess the maxillary branch of the trigeminal nerve by touching the lateral canthus and observing for a blink reflex. The mandibular branch is assessed by touching the base of the ear and observing a reflexive eyelid closure.

Head Tilt and Pathologic Nystagmus Observation (Cranial Nerve VIII)

The presence of a head tilt is best assessed when the animal's head is facing the examiner, by pulling an imaginary line through both eyes. The line should be horizontal. If a pathologic nystagmus is observed with the head at rest, its direction should be noted. The fast phase of the nystagmus is usually directed away from the side of the lesion. The head should then be elevated and the eyes observed for induction of a positional nystagmus or a change in the direction of the nystagmus. An important function of CN VIII is to maintain a normal head position that is parallel to a horizontal line.

Food Prehension (Cranial Nerve XII) and Masticatory Movement and Muscles (Cranial Nerve V)

The masticatory muscles are palpated for symmetry and atrophy. Unilateral involvement is represented by ipsilateral atrophy, whereas bilateral involvement leads to a dropped jaw. The animal should be offered food and the mastication observed. As the tongue is often used for prehension in ruminants, CN XII is also evaluated. If not, pull the tongue out of the mouth and observe the tongue for deviation and atrophy. In patients with a unilateral lesion of the hypoglossal nerve, the tongue will often fall from the mouth toward the lesion side.

Dysphagia and Laryngeal Problems (Cranial Nerve IX, Cranial Nerve X)

Cranial nerves IX and X are evaluated as a functional unit. Their abnormalities are disclosed on observation alone. Airway compromise (larynx) leads to difficulty breathing, dyspnea (noisy respirations), snoring, and voice change. Pharyngeal problems lead to dysphagia clinically characterized by choking, gagging, drooling from an inability to swallow saliva, and food coming out of the nostrils.

STEP 3: GAIT AND POSTURE

If the animal can stand safely, it should be allowed to walk freely in an enclosed area. The animal is walked at a slow pace, back and forth, in the direction of the examiner. The clinician should observe the front limb gait as the animal approaches and the hind limb gait as the animal walks away. Particular attention is given to the foot placement as the animal turns or changes direction and speed. A series of questions are then answered.

- Is the animal able to walk?
- Is the gait normal, symmetric, consistent?
- Is there postural abnormality: hunching of the back, low head carriage, or opisthotonus?

- Which limbs are affected (one limb, both hind limbs, the hind and front limbs, or the ipsilateral limbs)?
- Do the limbs circumduct or abduct during turns?
- Do the limbs interfere or knuckle during locomotion?

A particular question deserving a bit more attention is the possible presence of ataxia.

There are 3 types of ataxia: vestibular, cerebellar, and proprioceptive.

Vestibular Ataxia

Unilateral vestibular ataxia is ALWAYS associated with *a head tilt*, hypermetra, and hypertonia. The animal with a unilateral cerebellar lesion leans, falls, or turns on itself toward the side the head is tilted. With bilateral vestibular dysfunction, the head tilt is subtle on the more affected side but usually present. However, there is an intentional head tremor.

Cerebellar Ataxia

Strength is preserved and there are no proprioceptive deficits. The ascending proprioceptive pathways from the limbs to the cerebrum and the descending motor pathways (upper motor neurons) from the cerebrum to the limbs are intact. Consequently with cerebellar ataxia, there are no proprioceptive deficits (no knuckling) or weakness.

Proprioceptive Ataxia

Proprioceptive ataxia is also called spinal ataxia because it is usually observed with spinal cord disease. Proprioceptive ataxia is secondary to damage of the ascending proprioceptive pathways.

There is always a concomitant weakness because of the simultaneous involvement of the descending motor pathways. It is the concomitant presence of weakness that helps in differentiating this ataxia from the cerebellar ataxia. It is the most difficult of the 3 types of ataxia to recognize, especially in its early stage. Ruling out the two others is often easier.

Observing the cerebrospinal axis in relation to the foot placement while the animal walks freely, puts its head down to sniff, elevates its head to look around while walking, or changes direction are all great ways at evaluating proprioception. The animal can also be made to circle or be pulled by the tail while the examiner observes the foot placement. Moreover, lower motor neuron deficits are present in the gait. In the cow, gait observation is the only suitable way to evaluate for the presence of proprioceptive deficits or lower motor neuron disease.

STEP 4: POSTURAL REACTIONS

The postural reactions complement the evaluation of the gait. Their usefulness is best in identifying asymmetry between sides and front and hind limbs. Proprioceptive positioning, if done appropriately, evaluates proprioception.

Position the limb in an awkward position, one that should be immediately corrected. This test cannot be performed in an uncooperative or an aggressive animal. The examiner should determine the symmetry of any abnormality. The test results are not always easy to interpret. Keeping detailed notes on the observations and repeating the test may be one way to be confident that the conclusion is solid.

STEP 5: SPINAL REFLEXES

Flexor and extensor reflexes are evaluated for the front and the hind limbs. The spinal reflexes are examined with the animal in lateral recumbency, the side being evaluated in the upper position. Although easier on smaller-sized animals, it is worth trying even on adult cattle, especially if the animal is recumbent.

Extensor Reflex of the Front Limb

The extensor reflexes of the front limb assess the radial nerves and are evaluated by observing weight bearing on either of the front limbs. The radial nerve innervates the triceps muscles and the digit extensors. Cattle with radial nerve dysfunction walk on the dorsal aspect of the fetlock and, depending on the level of the lesion, may have a dropped elbow. Traumatic soft tissue ulcers occur if the animal is allowed to walk on its affected limb. If the animal is down, the extensor reflex is evaluated by observing if extensor tone can be solicited in the limb. This evaluation is done putting a hand under the foot of the animal and pushing the limb gently toward the animal until extensor tone appears.

The Patellar Reflex

The patellar reflex evaluates the motor and some of the sensory components of the femoral nerve. The femoral nerve innervates the flexor muscles of the hips and the extensor muscles of the stifle. It is the nerve responsible for weight bearing in the hind limb. The patellar reflex is a tendinous monosynaptic reflex.

Elicit the reflex by tapping the patellar tendon, and observe an extension of the stifle. The limb should be in a relaxed semiflexion. The flexion should be just enough so the tendon is tight. The tendon is first palpated. Then while keeping the fingers on the tendon, the limb is flexed until the tendon feels tight. It helps increase tension in the tendon to put a hand under the foot while extending the digits. The tapping on the tendon is done with a pendulum motion. If the limb is tense, the reflex will not be elicited. The strength of the reflex is proportional to the force applied to the tendon. The position of the limb is characteristic in lower motor neuron disease of the femoral nerve: the animal walks, dragging the limb behind and is unable to bear weight on the limb. As the limb is bearing more weight, the stifle joint collapses.

The Withdrawal (Flexor) Reflexes

In the front limbs, the flexor reflex evaluates the axillary, median, and ulnar nerves. In the hind limb, the reflex evaluates the motor part of the sciatic nerve, except for the hip flexion, which is controlled by the femoral nerve. The sensory function of the lateral part of the limb is provided by the sciatic nerve and the medial part by the femoral nerve. Consequently, for the flexor reflex to occur, the sensory part of both nerves, femoral and sciatic, must be intact.

The flexor reflex is examined by pinching (a hemostat is often necessary in order to elicit a reliable reflex response) the lateral digit while observing a flexion of the limb, and then the skin over the medial digit is pinched and the examiner observes again for a flexion of the limb. Because of the secondary myopathy from prolonged recumbency, flexor reflexes may be difficult to interpret. With loss of the lower motor neurons to the limb, there is weak or absence of flexion of one or more joints. In upper motor neuron disease, the joints flex but the overall strength with which this is done may be decreased.

The Muscle Tone

The limbs should be passively flexed and extended if possible. Animals with lower motor neuron disease have hypotonia or atonia and, by 1 week, neurogenic atrophy. The muscle mass should be evaluated for symmetry. In upper motor neuron disease, the tone is normal if the disease is mild or increased in marked or severe cases. Spasticity is best evaluated in small ruminants or in calves with the animal recumbent.

The Perineal Reflex

The perineal region is delineated by a change in the growth of the hair surrounding the anus. This reflex is assessed by gently touching, with a finger or a cotton swab, the perineal region under the animal's tail. Avoid manipulating the tail because this will cause a contraction of the anus preventing the examiner to assess the sensory part of the reflex because the anus is already contracted.

Test the reflexes on both sides of the body. The expected response is a downward contraction of the tail and an accompanying anal sphincter contraction, which may be hidden by the tail. Performed in this manner, the afferent limb of the reflex is the sensory part of the pudendal nerve, whereas the efferent limb consists of the caudal nerves. To evaluate the motor part of the pudendal nerve, a rectal examination observing for anal sphincter strength is preferable.

The Cutaneous Trunci Reflex

Multiple stimulations may be needed in order to induce this reflex in normal animals. Afferents in spinal nerves carry the impulse to the eighth cervical and first thoracic spinal segments by way of the spinal cord white matter. The impulses created by pinching the skin on one side ascend the spinal cord bilaterally. The efferent limb is the lateral thoracic nerve, which causes the skin to flinch. The reflex is elicited by pinching the skin with a hemostat, from the level of the wing of the ilium to T2, approximately 1 to 2 in on either side of the dorsal processes. The reflex is evaluated on both sides of the body. If the reflex is present at the wings of the ilium, there is no need to assess its presence any further along the animal's back because the afferent limb must be intact all the way in order to allow the contraction of the cutaneous trunci muscles by the lateral thoracic nerve (which originates from the C8 and T1 spinal segments but mainly from C8). The lesion is 1 to 4 vertebras above the site where the reflex returns.

STEP 6: PAIN PERCEPTION (NOCICEPTION)

The patients' conscious response to pain is evaluated at the end of the examination in order to maintain the their cooperation. With experience, one realizes that pain perception does not always need to be assessed because many clues are gleaned during the examination to inform the clinician as to the presence of pain perception. Because of the nature of our patients, the expressions *deep* and *superficial* pain should probably not be used in veterinary medicine. There is decreased, increased, or absence of pain perception.

SUMMARY

The neurologic examination of the ruminant is very much an exercise in observation. Even if intimidating at times, one should always perform the examination when pertinent and keep good notes of all the observations. As the clinician's expertise develops, the examination becomes fun to perform and the challenge of lesion localization is greatly facilitated.

REFERENCES

1. de Lahunta A, Glass E, Kent M. Veterinary neuroanatomy and clinical neurology. 4th edition. St Louis (MO): Elsevier-Saunders; 2015. p. 304–7.
2. Mayhew IGJ. Large animal neurology. 2nd edition. Oxford (United Kingdom): Wiley-Blackwell; 2008. p. 11–47.

Diagnostics and Ancillary Tests of Neurologic Dysfunction in the Ruminant

Dusty W. Nagy, DVM, MS, PhD

KEYWORDS

- Cerebrospinal fluid analysis • Radiography • Myelography • Computed tomography
- MRI

KEY POINTS

- Cerebrospinal fluid is good for helping determine the broad category of disease but will rarely provide a definitive diagnosis in ruminants with neurologic dysfunction.
- Animal size and financial limitations often limit our use of diagnostic imaging modalities.
- Radiography, myelography, computed tomography, and MRI have all been used successfully to aid in lesion localization and diagnosis of ruminant neurologic diseases.

DIFFERENTIATING NON–CENTRAL NERVOUS SYSTEM LESIONS

Symptoms associated with neurologic disease can occur from lesions within the central nervous system (CNS) or peripheral nervous system or several conditions that originate outside of the nervous system. Therefore, a variety of diagnostics can be used to help further characterize the disease process. Complete blood count and serum chemistry panel have little utility in diagnosis of CNS lesions. However, animals with hypocalcemia or metabolic acidemia may have changes in mentation consistent with cortical neurologic disease. In these cases serum calcium concentration, total carbon dioxide, or blood pH may help diagnose these conditions. Serum sodium concentrations may aid in the diagnosis of sodium chloride intoxication, depending on the stage of disease. Serum magnesium concentrations may help diagnose animals with hypomagnesemic tetany.

In addition, some deficiencies and toxicities may lead to structural lesions within the CNS but not reliably change the composition of the cerebrospinal fluid (CSF). In these cases specific assays for the compound of interest, such as vitamin A, copper, or lead, may aid in the diagnosis of disease.

The author has nothing to disclose.
Department of Veterinary Medicine and Surgery, College of Veterinary Medicine, University of Missouri, 900 East Campus Drive, Columbia, MO 65211, USA
E-mail address: nagyd@missouri.edu

Vet Clin Food Anim 33 (2017) 9–18
http://dx.doi.org/10.1016/j.cvfa.2016.09.002   **vetfood.theclinics.com**
0749-0720/17/© 2016 Elsevier Inc. All rights reserved.

DIAGNOSTICS FOR CENTRALLY LOCATED LESIONS
Cerebrospinal Fluid

Analysis of CSF is one of the most commonly performed ancillary diagnostic tests in ruminant species when investigating the cause of neurologic symptoms. It is rarely diagnostic, but, in conjunction with history and examination findings, aids in the differentiation of the broad category of diseases and narrowing of the differential diagnosis list. Changes in protein concentration, cell count, and differential can help differentiate inflammatory/infectious, neoplastic, parasitic, metabolic, and degenerative disease processes. In addition, some disease conditions with primary lesions outside of the CNS can mimic neurologic disease. Changes in CSF composition can help the veterinary practitioner remove these diseases from the differential list.

Collection

Collection of CSF is most often attempted at the lumbosacral (LS) space. The atlanto-occipital (AO) space can be used in ruminants but typically requires general anesthesia to achieve the head position necessary for a blind tap. In addition, the potential to damage vital structures is far greater at the AO space. Recently, AO CSF collection under sedation on a tilt table using ultrasound guidance has been described.[1] This study found the procedure to be quick and effective at obtaining high-quality AO samples for analysis. Despite this advance, in most instances, there is not a significant enough difference in sample composition based on collection site to warrant the increased risk associated with an AO tap. Studies that have compared LS with AO CSF composition in sheep have found no significant difference in CSF composition.[2,3] The main exception is in cases of spinal or epidural abscess whereby protein from the LS collection site is significantly higher than that from the AO site.

Collection of CSF at the LS space can be done standing in most animals, given that an adequate chute or stock is available for restraint. In recumbent animals or small ruminants that cannot be adequately restrained standing, sternal recumbency with the hips flexed forward is an alternative for positioning. The hip flexion expands the LS space, making access easier. This position also limits kicking and the need to specifically restrain the hind legs.[4] Successful collection of CSF from any location requires appropriate understanding of and attention to the bony landmarks.

The LS space is located along the dorsal midline caudal to L6, cranial to the sacrum, and medial to the cranial point on the sacral tuberosities. A depression along the dorsal midline can typically be palpated at the LS space. In mature cattle, a 4-in spinal needle will be required, whereas in small ruminants and camelids, a 2-in needle should provide adequate depth. Lambs and kids should only require a 1-in needle in length.[5] Ideally, the needle hub will be close to the skin during collection. This location will allow for better stabilization and less risk of trauma during the collection.

The animal should be clipped and prepared in surgical fashion. Sterile gloves should be used. Local analgesia can be provided using 1 to 2 mL lidocaine. In fractious animals, light sedation using xylazine or a low-dose ketamine/xylazine/butorphanol combination can be used to improve patient compliance.[6]

The needle is passed perpendicular to the spinal cord at a slight angle with the bevel facing the head. The needle will pass through skin and subcutaneous tissue followed by the interarcuate ligament and finally the meninges. Slight changes in resistance can be felt as the needle passes into different tissue planes. A pop is sometimes appreciated as the needle moves out of the interarcuate ligament. Some animals will move slightly or swish their tail when the meninges is penetrated. When the needle is in the subarachnoid space, CSF will well into the hub of the needle once the stylet is removed. Attention to landmarks and changes in needle resistance during passage is critical to successful CSF collection. Only 1 to 2 mL of CSF is required for analysis. Slow removal with minimal vacuum (1–2 mL) placed on the collection syringe will decrease the likelihood of trauma associated with collection.

Analysis

CSF protein concentration and cytologic examination are the cornerstones of CSF analysis in ruminant species (**Table 1**). Sodium and magnesium may be evaluated in cases whereby sodium chloride intoxication or hypomagnesemic tetany are suspected.[7,8] Additional evaluations may include specific gravity, glucose, lactate dehydrogenase, alkaline phosphatase sodium, potassium, chloride, and creatine kinase (**Table 2**). Although normal values are available for these analytes in cattle, they are not well evaluated or routinely used in the analysis of ruminant CSF.[9,10]

Cells within the CSF degenerate rapidly, necessitating immediate analysis. Storage in 11% autologous serum can preserve samples at 4°C for up to 24 hours with reasonable preservation of cellular architecture.[11] In this study cytologic agreement in fresh versus stored samples was better for animals with a neutrophilic pleocytosis (100%) than those with a mononuclear pleocytosis (70%).

CSF should be clear and colorless. The presence of turbidity suggests an elevated cell count. Cell count must be extremely high to generate turbidity visible to the naked eye. Animals can have significant elevations in cell count without obvious turbidity in the CSF. Reddish tinge to the CSF may indicate the presence of blood that could be from traumatic puncture or previous bleeding into the CNS. Xanthochromia, yellowing of the CSF, may be present because of the release of pigments after erythrocyte lysis within the CNS. Xanthochromia may be evident within 2 to 6 hours of a CNS bleeding event and may remain for up to 10 days.[12]

CSF protein concentration reliably increases with infectious and compressive conditions. In a study in sheep, no significant increase in CSF protein concentration was seen with toxic, metabolic, or traumatic causes. Animals with scrapie and polioencephalomalacia also showed no increase in CSF protein concentrations.[2] The prognostic ability of CSF protein has yet to be proven in ruminant species. One study found a trend toward survival in *Listeria*-infected sheep with low CSF protein concentrations when compared with those with higher concentrations.[2] This finding has not held true in subsequent work.[13]

Protein electrophoresis patterns in both normal and diseased sheep and cattle have been documented. However, the electrophoretic patterns do not seem to add significant information to the analysis of CSF over protein content alone.[14,15]

Cell count and differential have been evaluated for a variety of common ruminant neurologic diseases. A neutrophilic pleocytosis is most common in bacterial inflammatory diseases. In cases of meningoencephalitis and leptomeningitis in both cattle and lambs, neutrophil count reliably increases well more than the normal range.[4,16] Monocytic pleocytosis is most common with viral causes. It is also regularly present in cattle with listeriosis and has been documented in calves with otitis media interna.[17,18] Eosinophilic pleocytosis has been associated with parasitic diseases of the CNS, such as aberrant parasite migration in camelids and goats as well as coenurosis is sheep.[2,19,20]

Culture

Studies evaluating culture of the CSF present variable results. In calves with bacterial meningoencephalitis, culture of the CSF will often yield positive results.[4] However, a study in sheep found very few meningoencephalitis cases yielded a positive culture.[16]

Table 1
Cerebrospinal fluid values for normal and diseased cattle and sheep

	WBC ×10⁶/L	Protein (mg/dL)	Neutrophils (%)	Monocytes (%)	Lymphocytes (%)	Eosinophils (%)	Reference
Normal calves	3.0 (0–10)	15.9 (11–33)	4.3 (0–34)	38.26 (28.0–66.2)	57.39 (33.8–71.0)	0.05 (0–0.5)	St. Jean et al,[10] 1997
Normal adult cattle	<5	43	<5	—	>95	—	Scott et al,[15] 1990
Meningoencephalitis calf (median/range)	240 (5–1260)	316 (95–710)	83 (63–100)	4 (0–29)	0.5 (0–20)	—	Scott & Pennyk,[4] 1993
Cattle *Listeria* (median/range)	30 (1–332)	67 (21–141)	—	Reported as primarily large mononuclear cells and lymphocytes			Rebhun & deLahunta,[17] 1982
Normal sheep	11 (0–29)	23 (7–39)	45.7 (32–60)	29.2 (8.0–50.4)	21.4 (3.3–39.6)	0	Scott,[2] 1992
Sheep *Listeria* (median/range)	200 (12–250)	100 (50–280)	53 (0–100)	10 (0–72)	15 (0–50)	—	Scott,[13] 1993
Sheep meningitis (mean/range)	209 (0–539)	160 (70–250)	59.9 (35.1–84.7)	21.4 (0.8–42.0)	20.3 (4.6–36.0)	0	Scott,[2] 1992
Sheep polio (mean/range)	8 (2–14)	20 (5–35)	24 (10.8–37.2)	4 (0–11.5)	68.4 (47.2–89.6)	2 (0–6)	Scott,[2] 1992
Sheep spinal abscess (mean/range)	22 (12–32)	268 (227–309)	1.5	26	16.5	27	Scott,[2] 1992

Abbreviation: WBC, white blood cell.
Data from Refs.[2,4,10,13,15,17]

Table 2
Values for various cerebrospinal fluid analytes

Analyte	Mean	SD	SEM	Range	Collection Site	Reference
Glucose (mmol/L)	3.3	0.41	—	3.003–4.24	AO	St. Jean et al,[10] 1997
Creatine kinase (U/L)	2.17	1.21	—	0–4	AO	St. Jean et al,[10] 1997
Sodium (mEq/L)	137.27	1.77	—	134–139	AO	St. Jean et al,[10] 1997
Potassium (mEq/L)	2.88	0.07	—	2.8–3.0	AO	St. Jean et al,[10] 1997
Chloride (mEq/L)	123.17	1.77	—	121–126	AO	St. Jean et al,[10] 1997
Calcium (mmol/L)	1.5	0.035	—	1.45–1.55	AO	St. Jean et al,[10] 1997
Phosphorus (mmol/L)	0.462	0.039	—	0.42–0.52	AO	St. Jean et al,[10] 1997
Alkaline phosphatase (U/L)	1.67	0.75	—	1–3	AO	St. Jean et al,[10] 1997
Urea (mmol/L)	2.08	0.43	—	1.43–2.5	AO	St. Jean et al,[10] 1997
Creatinine (mmol/L)	54.8	6.19	—	44.2–61.9	AO	St. Jean et al,[10] 1997
Specific gravity	1.0056	0.00049	—	1.005–1.006	AO	St. Jean et al,[10] 1997
Creatine kinase (U/L)	11.438	—	3.431	2–48	LS	Welles et al,[9] 1992
Glucose (mg/dL)	42.875	—	0.991	37–51	LS	Welles et al,[9] 1992
Magnesium (mEq/L)	1.988	—	0.026	1.8–2.1	LS	Welles et al,[9] 1992
Protein (mg/dL)	39.163	—	3.389	23.4–66.3	LS	Welles et al,[9] 1992
Lactate dehydrogenase (U/L)	13.938	—	1.318	2–25	LS	Welles et al,[9] 1992
Sodium (mmol/L)	140	—	0.780	132–142	LS	Welles et al,[9] 1992
Potassium (mmol/L)	2.956	—	0.030	2.7–3.2	LS	Welles et al,[9] 1992
Osmolality (mOsm/kg)	285.813	—	2.199	272–300	LS	Welles et al,[9] 1992

Abbreviations: SD, standard deviation; SEM, standard error of mean.

Data from Welles EG, Tyler JW, Sorjonen DC, et al. Composition and analysis of cerebrospinal fluid in clinically normal adult cattle. Am J Vet Res 1992;53:2050–56; and St. Jean G, Yvorchuk-St. Jean K, Anderson DE, et al. Cerebrospinal fluid constituents collected at the atlanto-occipital site of xylazine hydrochloride sedated, healthy 8-week-old Holstein calves. Can J Vet Res 1997;61:108–12.

Studies specifically attempting to culture *Listeria* from clinical cases also demonstrate poor recovery of the organism from both cattle and sheep.[21] In addition to the varying ability to culture organisms, the time to generate culture and antimicrobial sensitivity data versus the duration of neurologic disease in many ruminants often limits the utility of antemortem culture of the CSF.

Diagnostic Imaging

Diagnostic imaging is common in small animal and human medicine for patients with neurologic dysfunction. The use of these modalities is less common in ruminant species, partially because of cost and in some cases size limitations of the equipment. In addition, the literature on the use and outcome interpretation of these modalities is often lacking for ruminant species. Despite this, the evolution of pet-quality and high-dollar reproductive animals is generating a niche for the use of these modalities in ruminant patients.

Ultrasonography

Ultrasound uses high-frequency sound waves to generate an image. A sound wave is emitted from the transducer into the area of interest on a patient. The wave will pass through body tissues at a variable rate and depth depending on tissue density. A portion will be returned to the transducer, and the rate at which it is returned will be translated into a visible image. Shorter wavelengths (higher frequency) generate more detailed images, but longer wavelengths (lower frequency) penetrate deeper into patients. Both air and bone pose significant barriers to sound wave propagation.

The use of ultrasonography in ruminant neurologic disease has not been heavily used. The inability of sound waves to effectively penetrate bone limits the use in neurologic disease. The use of ultrasound has been described to aid in needle placement for AO CSF collection.[1] It has also been described as an aid in differentiating meningocele from meningoencephalocele and as diagnostic tool in calves with peripheral vestibular signs suspected of having otitis media/interna.[18,22]

Radiography/Myelography

Radiography uses a beam of ionizing radiation to generate an image. The differential absorption of the x-rays by body tissues generates a 2-dimensional image on a capture substrate. In older systems, x-rays are passed through patients and onto a film cassette that captures the image. Once processed this can be viewed and interpreted using a backlight system. Newer computed radiography systems use imaging plates that contain photostimulatable phosphors that can store the x-ray energy. The plate is then scanned and a digital image is generated. Direct or digital radiography systems use either a flat panel detector or digital cassette to capture the x-rays passed through patients, which is immediately converted to a digital image that can often be viewed patient side, depending on the system setup.

Because of the summation of tissues when generating a radiographic image and the large body size of many ruminants, plain radiographs are most useful in cases that involve bone. Spinal fracture, luxation, and osteomyelitis can be seen radiographically depending on the size of the animal. Smaller portable systems may have trouble imaging cattle but may still provide adequate images in calves, small ruminants, and camelids. In cattle, a cervical fracture may be found using machines with ample power. However, the size of a mature cow limits the efficacy of radiographs when attempting to image thoracic or lumbar spine. Plain radiographs have little utility in diagnosing parenchymal diseases of the spinal cord or brain.

Radiography has been used to aid in the diagnosis of ruminant neurologic diseases whereby bony abnormalities are the prominent abnormality causing the clinical signs. In sheep it has been used to diagnose vertebral body malformations and malalignments. Clinical signs were well correlated to the radiographic abnormalities in the spine and the expected affected spinal cord segments.[23,24] In an additional case in a Boer goat, survey radiographs were suggestive of discospondylitis and possible vertebral fracture.[25]

Myelography is the addition of a contrast media to the subarachnoid space to enhance images obtained by radiography or potentially computed tomography (CT). This imaging may highlight pathologies that were not readily detectible without the presence of the contrast media. Myelography can be used to aid in the diagnosis of dynamic or static compressive lesions of the spinal cord or space-occupying lesions within the spinal canal as the addition of contrast highlights these defects. Myelography requires general anesthesia and the capability to move and adjust positioning of the animal.

Radiographic myelography has been reported in sheep and calves for aid in diagnosis of cervical spinal cord disease.[26,27] In 2 calves with spinal epidural abscesses, thinning of the dye line or failure of contrast media progression were found to be suggestive of a space-occupying lesion.[26] In one calf with complete attenuation of the dye line, severe bony abnormalities were present and documented on survey radiographs. The other calf had no radiographic changes evident on survey films and only mild attenuation of the dye line. In this calf, advanced imaging was required to completely elucidate the extent of the lesion. In sheep with compressive cervical myelopathy, radiographic myelography was able to determine lesion location in all animals imaged.[27]

Myelography clearly offers advantages over survey radiographs for localizing spinal cord lesions where bony abnormalities are not present. However, the variety of lesions seen in ruminant species that cause compressive spinal cord disease limit myelography's utility in definitive diagnosis of the disease process, and it is likely best suited to aid in lesion localization. In animals whereby euthanasia is the likely outcome if a lesion is present, radiographs and myelography may provide adequate information for less expense than advanced imaging modalities or when these modalities are unavailable.

Computed Tomography

Similar to radiography, CT uses the differential absorption of x-rays by body tissues to generate an image. The basis of the CT consists of the gantry, which holds the x-ray tube, and the table, which holds the patients. The tube emits a fan-shaped beam of x-rays that are picked up by an array of sensors within the gantry. The thickness of the beam is variable based on the machine. The thinner the beam, the more detail generated on the resulting image. During the scanning phase of the examination, the table moves patients through the gantry allowing for image acquisition. After which, the data generated are sent to the computer, which reconstructs the examination into a cross-sectional image of the patients. The ability to remove superimposing tissues allows for clearer, more accurate visualization of organ structure and location.

CT scans are extremely quick to run and can often be done under short-duration or injectable anesthetics in small ruminants and calves. This ability limits the overall anesthetic time and cost, particularly when compared with MRI. As a general rule, they are best used for cross-sectional imaging when bony involvement is expected. However, CT can be used effectively in some cases whereby the abnormality lies in soft tissue.

CT has been used for a variety of disease processes in small and large ruminants as well as camelid species. Bony lesions are uniformly found using CT.[27,28] It has been shown to be effective at locating space-occupying lesions, such as abscesses, cysts, hydrocephalus, and coenurosis lesions.[28–31] In addition, otitis media, discospondylitis, and malformations involving the cerebral cortex have also been found using CT.[22,28] In one retrospective study looking at the use of CT in cattle disease, most neurologic cases were identified. In this study, 7 cases presented for motor incoordination had no significant findings on CT. In 5 of these, lesions were also not diagnosable by histopathology suggesting that disease may be nonstructural in nature. One case was later found to have a brainstem abscess. In this case, the investigators hypothesized that beam-hardening artifacts made evaluation of the brainstem in cattle difficult. These findings suggest that CT is a viable imaging modality for cattle neurologic disease with the exception of brainstem lesions.

MRI

Similar to CT, MRI generates a cross-sectional image of patients. However, unlike radiography and CT, MRI does not use ionizing radiation and is, thus, safer for patients. An MRI uses magnets to alter the alignment of the water molecules within the body. The changes in the alignment are detected by the scanner and then converted to a 3-dimensional cross-sectional image by the computer. This modality does an exceptional job at highlighting differences in soft tissue planes. Therefore, it is often chosen when imaging the brain and spinal cord when subtleties in soft tissues need to be elucidated. Unlike CT, MRI scans are long and will require general anesthesia with prolonged down time for the animal.

Despite the lack of timeliness and cost, case reports and studies using MRI on ruminants are appearing in the literature with increasing frequency. There are cases supporting its use for the diagnosis of spinal epidural abscess and brainstem abscess in calves as well as cortical abscess and cerebellar abiotrophy in goats.[26,32–34] A research study looking at sheep as a model for Creutzfeldt-Jakob disease found diffuse cerebral atrophy in both symptomatic and asymptomatic sheep infected with scrapie.[35]

Electrodiagnostic Tests

A variety of electrodiagnostic tests have been used in cattle and sheep.[36–38] In sheep, they are most often conducted under research settings as a model of human disease. Currently, encephalography is most often used as an evaluative tool in surgical pain or humane slaughter studies.[39,40] The complexity of conducting and interpreting these diagnostic tests limits their usage to academic settings. The lack of normal data in health and disease also severely limits their utility in clinical practice.

REFERENCES

1. Braun U, Attiger J, Brammertz C. Ultrasonographic examination of the spinal cord and collection of cerebrospinal fluid from the atlanto-occipital space in cattle. BMC Vet Res 2015;11:227–33.
2. Scott PR. Analysis of cerebrospinal fluid from field cases of some common ovine neurological diseases. Br Vet J 1992;148:15–22.
3. Scott PR, Will RG. A report of Froin's syndrome in five ovine thoracolumbar epidural abscess cases. Br Vet J 1991;147:582–4.
4. Scott PR, Penny CD. A field study of meningoencephalitis in calves with particular reference to analysis of cerebrospinal fluid. Vet Rec 1993;133:119–21.
5. Scott PR. The collection and analysis of cerebrospinal fluid as an aid to diagnosis in ruminant neurological disease. Br Vet J 1995;151:603–14.
6. Abrahamsen EJ. Chemical restraint and injectable anesthesia of ruminants. Vet Clin North Am Food Anim Pract 2013;29:209–27.
7. Pearson EG, Kallfelz FA. A case of presumptive salt poisoning (water deprivation) in veal calves. Cornell Vet 1982;72:142–9.
8. McCoy MA, Hutchinson T, Davison G, et al. Postmortem biochemical markers of experimentally induced hypomagnesaemic tetany in cattle. Vet Rec 2001;148:268–73.
9. Welles EG, Tyler JW, Sorjonen DC, et al. Composition and analysis of cerebrospinal fluid in clinically normal adult cattle. Am J Vet Res 1992;53:2050–6.
10. St. Jean G, Yvorchuk-St. Jean K, Anderson DE, et al. Cerebrospinal fluid constituents collected at the atlanto-occipital site of xylazine hydrochloride sedated, healthy 8-week-old Holstein calves. Can J Vet Res 1997;61:108–12.
11. Bellino C, Miniscalco B, Bertone I, et al. Analysis of cerebrospinal fluid from cattle with central nervous system disorders after storage for 24 hours with autologous serum. BMC Vet Res 2015;11:201–5.

12. Mayhew IG, Beal CR. Techniques of analysis of cerebrospinal fluid. Vet Clin North Am Small Anim Pract 1980;10:155–76.

13. Scott PR. A field study of ovine listerial meningo-encephalitis with particular reference to cerebrospinal fluid analysis as an aid to diagnosis and prognosis. Br Vet J 1993;149:165–70.

14. Scott PR. Total protein and electrophoretic pattern of cerebrospinal fluid in sheep with some common neurological disorders. Cornell Vet 1993;83:199–204.

15. Scott PR, Aldridge BM, Clarke M, et al. Cerebrospinal fluid studies in normal cows and cases of bovine spongiform encephalopathy. Br Vet J 1990;146:88–90.

16. Scott PR, Sargison ND, Penny CD, et al. A field study of ovine meningoencephalitis. Vet Rec 1994;135:154–6.

17. Rebhun WC, deLahunta A. Diagnosis and treatment of bovine listeriosis. J Am Vet Med Assoc 1982;180:395–8.

18. Bernier-Gosselin V, Francoz D, Babkine M, et al. A retrospective study of 29 cases of otitis media/interna in dairy calves. Can Vet J 2012;53:957–62.

19. Baumgartner W, Zajac A, Hull BL, et al. Parelaphostrongylosis in llamas. J Am Vet Med Assoc 1985;187:1243–5.

20. Kopcha M, Marteniuk JV, Sills R, et al. Cerebrospinal nematodiasis in a goat herd. J Am Vet Med Assoc 1989;194:1439–42.

21. Peters M, Pohlenz J, Jaton K, et al. Studies of the detection of Listeria monocytogenes by culture and PCR in cerebrospinal fluid samples from ruminants with listeric encephalitis. Zentralbl Veterinarmed B 1995;42:84–8.

22. Ohba Y, Iguchi T, Hirose Y, et al. Computer tomography diagnosis of meningoencephalocele in a calf. J Vet Med Sci 2008;70:829–31.

23. Hill BD, O'Dempsey ND, Carlisle CH. Cervicothoracic vertebral subluxation causing ataxia in sheep. Aust Vet J 1993;70:156–7.

24. Lakritz J, Barr BC, George LW, et al. Cervical and thoracic vertebral malformation ("weak neck") in Colombia lambs. J Vet Intern Med 1995;9:393–8.

25. Levine GJ, Bissett WT, Cole RC, et al. Imaging diagnosis-bacterial diskospondylitis in a goat. Vet Radiol Ultrasound 2006;47:585–8.

26. Zani DD, Romano L, Scandella M, et al. Spinal epidural abscess in two calves. Vet Surg 2008;37:801–8.

27. Penny C, Macrae A, Hagen R, et al. Compressive cervical myelopathy in young Texel and Beltex sheep. J Vet Intern Med 2007;21:322–7.

28. Lee K, Yamada Y, Tsuneda R, et al. Clinical experience of using multidetector-row CT for the diagnosis of disorders in cattle. Vet Rec 2009;165:559–62.

29. El-Khodery S, Yamada K, Aoki D, et al. Brain abscess in a Japanese Black calf: utility of computed tomography (CT). J Vet Med Sci 2008;70:727–30.

30. Gonzalo-Orden JM, Diez A, Altonaga JR, et al. Computed tomographic findings in ovine coenurosis. Vet Radiol Ultrasound 1999;40:441–4.

31. Hardefeldt LA, Rylander H, Iskandar BJ, et al. Diagnosis and surgical treatment of an intracranial cyst in an alpaca cria. J Am Vet Med Assoc 2012;240:1501–6.

32. Tsuka T, Taura Y. Abscess of bovine brain stem diagnosed by contrast MRI examinations. J Vet Med Sci 1999;61:425–7.

33. Dennler M, Carrera I, Beckmann K, et al. Imaging diagnosis-conventional and functional magnetic resonance imaging of a brain abscess in a goat. Vet Radiol Ultrasound 2014;55:68–73.

34. Koehler JW, Newcomer BW, Holland M. A novel inherited cerebellar abiotrophy in a cohort of related goats. J Comp Pathol 2015;153:135–9.

35. McKnight AL, Minkoff LA, Sutton DL, et al. Generalized cerebral atrophy seen on MRI in a naturally exposed animal model for Creutzfeldt-Jakob disease. J Transl Med 2010;8:125–32.

36. Opdam HI, Federico P, Jackson GD, et al. A sheep model for the study of focal epilepsy with concurrent intracranial EEG and functional MRI. Epilepsia 2002;43: 779–87.

37. Cwynar P, Kolacz R, Walerjan P. Electroencephalographic recordings of physiological activity of the sheep cerebral cortex. Pol J Vet Sci 2014;17:613–23.

38. Takeuchi T, Sitizyo K, Harada E. Analysis of the electroencephalogram in growing calves by use of power spectrum and cross correlation. Am J Vet Res 1998;59: 777–81.

39. Gibson TJ, Johnson CB, Murrell JC, et al. Electroencephalographic responses to concussive non-penetrative captive-bolt stunning in halothane - anaesthetised calves. N Z Vet J 2009;57:90–5.

40. Dockweiler JC, Coetzee JF, Edwards-Callaway LN, et al. Effect of castration method on neurohormonal and electroencephalographic stress indicators in Holstein calves of different ages. J Dairy Sci 2013;96:4340–54.

Localization of Neurologic Lesions in Ruminants

Kevin E. Washburn, DVM

KEYWORDS

- Ruminant • Lesion localization • Neurologic deficits

KEY POINTS

- Localization of the origin of neurologic signs is vital to narrowing the differential list.
- Once the origin of clinical symptoms is discovered and the differential list is narrowed, further diagnostics can be more readily determined to arrive at a likely diagnosis.
- Determining the most likely diagnosis is critical because it guides prognosis and treatment regimens.
- Sometimes determining prognosis, herd ramifications, and zoonotic potential is economically and prudently more important than successful treatment and outcome.
- Although not always possible, give the animal 1 disease or condition that accounts for all clinical signs.

INTRODUCTION

The examination of a ruminant with neurologic dysfunction often presents many challenges to the diagnostician.[1–3] Challenges include the size of the animal, unruliness, economic constraints, an alarmed owner, and limited diagnostic tools that can practically be applied to the case. Therefore, the first step in these cases is to determine the most likely source of the neurologic symptoms so that an accurate prognosis and treatment regimen can be developed. There are myriad possible differentials for neurologic symptoms in ruminants that include truly primary neurologic disease, such as enzootic lymphosarcoma in the spinal canal, and secondary neurologic disease, such as hypomagnesemia. A thorough history and physical and neurologic examination are paramount to localization of the origin of neurologic signs. Once determined, the clinician can often use all the pieces of information gathered to arrive at a working diagnosis or narrowed differential list. Subsequently, it may then be possible to use only a few practical diagnostic tests, such as a cerebrospinal fluid

The author has no financial disclosures to provide.
Department of Large Animal Clinical Sciences, Food Animal Medicine, Texas A&M University, College of Veterinary Medicine and Biomedical Sciences, College Station, TX 77843, USA
E-mail address: kwashburn@cvm.tamu.edu

http://dx.doi.org/10.1016/j.cvfa.2016.09.003
0749-0720/17/© 2016 Elsevier Inc. All rights reserved.
vetfood.theclinics.com

analysis, to achieve a definitive diagnosis. This article categorizes and describes common clinical signs in ruminants localizable to various regions of the central nervous system to equip clinicians with the ability to more readily determine the origin(s) of neurologic dysfunction and proceed with more discriminating diagnostic tests if warranted. Furthermore, it is hoped that this categorization can be used as an aid in answering 2 fundamental questions: Is it rostral or caudal to the foramen magnum? and Is it primary or secondary neurologic disease?

CEREBRUM

Common clinical signs localizable to the cerebrum
Opisthotonus
Blindness (with an intact pupillary light reflex)
Abnormal mentation
Change in behavior
Aimless wandering or compulsive circling
Seizures
Abnormal vocalization

Opisthotonus

Opisthotonus is defined as dorsiflexion of the head and neck. If the animal is able to sit sternal, this is sometimes referred to as *stargazing*. In the author's experience, however, ruminants with opisthotonus more frequently lie in lateral recumbency and are unable to right themselves. Ruminants with advanced tetanus or hypomagnesemia may appear to have opisthotonus as well; therefore, it is important to assess the complete neurologic and physical examination findings to determine its origin.

Blindness

Vision can, in part, be assessed from a distance as the animal is asked to navigate unfamiliar surroundings. It is important, especially with small ruminants, to assess the animals as individuals because their strong herd instincts allow them to use other heightened senses and their herd mates to navigate their environment. A complete ocular neurologic examination should follow and aid the clinician in determining whether the lack of vision is of cerebral cortical origin. Lack of vision with an intact pupillary light reflex is a hallmark of cerebral cortical disease. If the pupillary light reflex is absent unilaterally or bilaterally, the clinician should consider dysfunction of the ocular pathways or retina (vitamin A deficiency).

Abnormal Mentation

Although abnormal mentation in a ruminant can range from stupor and depression to excitement and mania, the primary determinant is how the animal is responding to its environment. Although owners may consider this to be "behavior," the natural temperament of the animal can mimic abnormalities in mentation in some cases. It is straightforward to recognize the extreme in abnormal mentation; however, the author argues that often the alteration from the normal temperament of the animal is subtle. Consequently, abnormal mentation assessment should be coupled, if possible, with the caveat of whether a change has occurred.

Change in Behavior

Because abnormal mentation can often be normal for some individual animals due to temperament (ie, a normally fractious animal when confined may also be manic from an altered mentation), the author always quizzes the owner about changes from normal for that particular animal. Former exhibition animals are most often calm when handled; however, if the owner now notes that they are unusually unruly, it could be indicative of a change in behavior due to cerebral disease.

Aimless Wandering or Compulsive Circling

Without cerebral function, the brainstem takes over in locomotion, resulting in a slow, forward movement with no guidance from the cerebrum. When an animal reaches an obstacle or enclosure, if visual, the animal may press into it or circle away from it. If blind, the animal may circle an enclosure; however, if diffuse cerebral disease is present, this circling is in no particular direction.

Seizures

Seizures are involuntary episodes of muscular activity during which an animal becomes laterally recumbent with an altered mentation. The involuntary muscular activity usually results in paddling of the limbs. Time between episodes may be hours (early nervous coccidiosis) or minutes (polioencephalomalacia) depending on the cause. Ruminants in lateral recumbency with other conditions, such as advanced tetanus and hypomagnesemia, may appear to be having seizures; however, these animals do not have an altered mentation and are usually visual.

Abnormal Vocalization

Vocalization considered abnormal includes instances where vocalization is continuous, involuntary, and unstoppable by external stimuli. Furthermore, changes in pitch or volume during these episodes may indicate not only cerebral disease but also disease of the innervation to the pharyngeal region (rabies).

CEREBELLUM

Common clinical signs localizable to the cerebellum
Ataxia without weakness
Truncal sway
Hypermetria
Absent menace
Wide base stance
Intention tremors

Ataxia Without Weakness

Ataxia is abnormal gait with accompanying incoordination. The gait is controlled by the cerebellum, brainstem, spinal cord, and peripheral nerves. Determining whether the ataxia is of cerebellar dysfunction requires evaluating for the presence or absence of muscle strength. Strength can be assessed by pulling on the tail while the animal is moving in an attempt to pull it off course. The ability of the animal to resist this motion and apply strength to keep itself on course is indicative of normal muscle tone. This procedure may be impossible to perform safely on all cases. Observing the gait from a distance for proprioceptive deficits during ataxia can be helpful as well. Ruminants with cerebellar disease do not have proprioceptive deficits during ataxia.

Truncal Sway

Truncal sway is simply a side-to-side swaying of the body during forward locomotion. This can also be observed in animals with lesions in the cervical spinal cord.

Hypermetria

Hypermetria is an exaggerated movement of the limbs during forward movement. In ruminants, hypermetria is most easily and readily appreciated in the forelimbs.

Wide Base Stance

Although not specific for cerebellar disease, positioning the limbs further away from their normal axial plane can be indicative of cerebellar dysfunction. The loss of muscle coordination leads the animal to position itself such that it may maintain balance. In the opinion of the author, these animals appear to be "holding on" to the ground for fear of falling over.

Intention Tremors

Small, rapid muscle contractions in various muscle groups that occur when an animal is moving are referred to as *intention tremors*. A bobbing of the head up and down as the animal moves to drink or eat is an example of an intention tremor as are diffuse areas of small, rapid contractions occurring when the animal initiates movement. Tremors that occur at rest are much less likely of cerebellar origin.

VESTIBULAR SYSTEM

Localizing lesions of the vestibular system to either a peripheral or central lesion is important for determining the prognosis of some cases. In the author's experience, peripheral vestibular disease responds more favorably to treatment than does a central lesion (**Table 1**).

Head Tilt to the Side of the Lesion

A head tilt is defined as a continuous positioning of the head so that the eyes are off the horizontal plane and the muzzle of the animal is tilted away from the side of the lesion.

Table 1 Common clinical signs localizable to the vestibular system		
Clinical Sign	Peripheral (Cranial Nerve 8)	Central (Cranial Nerve 8 Brainstem Nuclei)
Head tilt to the side of the lesion	+	+
Falling/leaning/circling to the side of the lesion	+	+
Nystagmus	+/−	+
Proprioceptive deficits on the side of the lesion	−	+
Depression/anorexia	−	+

This condition is present with both peripheral and central cranial nerve VIII dysfunction; however, it is more severe and often accompanied by recumbency with central lesions.

Falling/Leaning/Circling to the Side of the Lesion

Falling, leaning, and circling to the side of the lesion occur with both peripheral and central lesions. Central lesions most often result, however, in smaller diameter circles, ultimately resulting in recumbency with the head turned into the flank on the side of the lesion.

Nystagmus

Lesions involving the vestibulocochlear nuclei often result in a sustained nystagmus. The nystagmus is typically horizontal but may change to vertical or rotary when the head position is changed. The fast phase is away from the side of the lesion.

Proprioceptive Deficits on the Side of the Lesion

Cattle with severe central lesions typically display proprioceptive deficits on the side of the lesion most readily observed in the forelimbs. The result of these deficits in a standing animal is extension of the forelimb opposite the side of the lesion.

Depression/Anorexia

Animals with signs of vestibular dysfunction that are also depressed and anorexic are most typical of a central lesion involving the brainstem nuclei and reticular activating system. These animals also are most likely to be recumbent and moribund.

CRANIAL NERVES

As the cranial nerves are examined, it is important to note that these nerves have either sensory, motor, or both modes of function. It is possible, therefore, to lose one functional aspect of a cranial nerve while the other remains intact (**Table 2**).

I Through IV

Cranial nerve I is difficult to evaluate effectively and is not discussed. Deficits in cranial nerve II are noted by blindness and absence of the pupillary light reflex. An absence of

Table 2 Cranial nerve modes of function	
Cranial Nerve	**Sensory, Motor, or Both**
I	Sensory
II	Sensory
III	Motor
IV	Motor
V	Both
VI	Motor
VII	Both
VIII	Sensory
IX	Both
X	Both
XI	Motor
XII	Motor

the pupillary light reflex, ventrolateral strabismus, and dilation of the pupils is typical of cranial nerve III dysfunction. Cranial nerve IV deficits are manifested as dorsomedial strabismus.

V Through VIII

Loss of sensation to the head and corneal surface is indicative of damage to cranial nerve V, as is a dropped, slack jaw. Deficits in cranial nerve VI are manifested as a ventromedial strabismus and an inability to retract the globe after a stimulus. Cranial nerve VII is motor to the muscles of the face, therefore, droopy ears, eyelids, and lips; deviation of the nasal filtrum (cattle do not display this sign); and inability to blink are signs of dysfunction. Cranial nerve VIII peripheral disorders create head tilt, circling, and leaning/falling to the side of the lesion.

IX Through XII

Cranial nerves IX and X disorders cause an inability to swallow. A flaccid protruding tongue with decreased or absent ability to retract it is indicative of cranial nerve XII disease. Cranial nerve XI is difficult to evaluate; however, an inability to turn the head and neck from side to side away from a noxious stimulus is suggestive of dysfunction (**Table 3**).

RETICULAR ACTIVATING SYSTEM, THALAMUS, HYPOTHALAMUS

Table 3 Clinical signs localizable to the reticular activating system, thalamus, and hypothalamus of the ruminant	
Depression/altered mentation	Reticular activating system
Difficulty regulating body temperature	Thalamus/hypothalamus
Depressed respiration	Reticular activating system

Depression/Altered Mentation

Lesions of the reticular activating system in the brainstem cause profound depression. Sometimes due to the normal demeanor of the animal, this may be a subjective assessment; however, when a change has occurred, determination of neurologically derived depression becomes more reliable.

Difficulty Regulating Body Temperature

Large variations in core body temperature without any evidence of an infectious cause should be considered as having lesions in the thalamus and/or hypothalamus. After heat stress, camelids and young calves can experience prolonged periods of decreased ability to regulate body temperature.

Depressed Respiration

The respiratory centers in the brainstem are controlled by the reticular activating system. Therefore, respiratory rate decreases in response to disease conditions.

SPINAL CORD
C1 to C5 Vertebrae

Altered head and neck movements with no cranial nerve abnormalities are often noted with lesions within this region of the spinal cord. Furthermore, all reflexes of the fore and hind limbs are exaggerated (hyperreflexia). The increased extensor tone noted in all limbs also results in ataxia with or without truncal sway. When pivoting, animals may display proprioceptive deficits in the pivot limb (inside limb). Severe cervical lesions cranial to C4 often result in lateral recumbency.

C6 to T2 Vertebrae

Ruminants with lesions from C6 to T2 display depressed to absent reflexes with decreased muscle tone in the forelimbs and exaggerated hind limb reflexes with normal muscle tone in the hind limbs. Knuckling, stumbling, and collapse of the fore-limbs are indicative of lower motor neuron disease.

T3 to L3 Vertebrae

Reflexes in the forelimbs are normal, whereas hind limb reflexes are exaggerated. Pro-prioceptive deficits are noted in the hind limbs in addition to ataxia. Larger ruminants may dog sit, even though muscle tone and extensor tone are increased.

L4 to L6 Vertebrae

The most notable clinical difference in ruminants with lesions further caudal in the lum-bar portions of the spinal cord is the absence of hind limb reflexes and decreased muscle tone. In larger ruminants, this clinically may be difficult to distinguish between lesions here and between T2 and L3. If practical, however, performing hind limb spinal reflexes and evaluating muscle tone should be differentiating.

S1 to S3 Vertebrae

Decreased anal tone, tail tone, and loss of sensation to the perineal region are typical of lesions in this region. Furthermore, a distended urinary bladder that dribbles constantly is indicative of a lower motor neuron urinary bladder lesion.

SUMMARY

Overall, with a proper history and physical and neurologic examination, signs of neuro-logic dysfunction can be localized to a primary or secondary origin. Once localized, clinicians can then answer the following questions: Is it primary neurologic disease? and Is it rostral or caudal to the foramen magnum? Determining the most likely origin greatly narrows the differential list, streamlines the number of ancillary tests neces-sary, greatly improves the accuracy of prognosis, and guides treatment regimens.

REFERENCES

1. de Lahunta A, Glass E, Kent M. Veterinary neuroanatomy and clinical neurology. 4th edition. St Louis: Elsevier-Saunders; 2015.
2. Mayhew IGJ. Large animal neurology. 2nd edition. Oxford: Wiley-Blackwell; 2008.
3. Constable PD. Clinical examination of the ruminant nervous system. Vet Clin North Am Food Anim Pract 2004;20:185–214.

Cerebral Disorders of Calves

Vincent Dore, DMV, MS, Geof Smith, DVM, MS, PhD*

KEYWORDS

- Hypernatremia • Sodium toxicity • Polioencephalomalacia • Meningitis • Neurology

KEY POINTS

- The most common causes of cerebral disorders in calves are polioencephalomalacia (PEM), bacterial meningitis (usually in calves less than 2–3 weeks of age), and hypernatremia (salt poisoning).
- PEM can be caused by several things, including thiamine deficiency and sulfur toxicity, as well as other dietary factors. Regardless of cause, thiamine supplementation is the treatment of choice in cattle suspected of having this disease.
- Bacterial meningitis generally occurs in calves less than 2 weeks of age as a sequelae of septicemia and failure of passive transfer. Treatment of meningitis is extremely difficult and, therefore, effort should be placed on prevention.
- Hypernatremia (salt poisoning) is becoming recognized more frequently in calves as related to ingestion of high sodium levels during treatment of diarrhea or possibly from ingestion of water with high sodium. Treatment requires careful attention to reduce sodium concentrations slowly over time to prevent the formation of cerebral edema.

 Video content accompanies this article at http://www.vetfood.theclinics.com.

Diseases affecting the forebrain or cerebrum are probably the most common neurologic conditions encountered in cattle. In general, clinical signs attributable to cerebral disease are characterized by abnormal mentation with a normal gait and posture. Clinical signs suggestive of abnormal mentation can include circling, blindness, mania, aggressive behavior, and seizure activity, along with what is often described as head pressing. The list of diseases that could cause cerebral disease in cattle is long and includes lead toxicity, polioencephalomalacia (PEM), bacterial meningitis, thromboembolic meningoencephalitis due to *Histophilus somni*, Bovine herpesvirus type 1, rabies, nervous coccidiosis, brain abscess, pseudorabies, urea toxicity, and malignant catarrhal fever. Also included are metabolic disturbances such as hypernatremia,

---

The authors have nothing to disclose.
Department of Population Health & Pathobiology, North Carolina State University, 1060 William Moore Drive, Raleigh, NC 27607, USA
* Corresponding author.
E-mail address: Geoffrey_Smith@ncsu.edu

hypocalcemia, hypomagnesemia, hypokalemia, hepatic encephalopathy, Vitamin A deficiency, and severe acid-base derangements.[1] Consideration of the signalment and history of the animal is critical when investigating neurologic disease. Several of the previously listed diseases could affect dairy or beef calves under 6 to 9 months of age. A brain abscess is always possible in young calves, although they are relatively uncommon. Typically, these would show a slow but progressive onset of clinical signs resulting from the space-occupying lesion in the cerebrum. Thromboembolic meningoencephalitis and nervous coccidiosis can also be seen in feedlot calves on occasion and warrant mention. However, the most common causes of cerebral disorders in calves are PEM, bacterial meningitis (usually in calves less than 2–3 weeks of age), and hypernatremia (salt poisoning). These are the primary focus of this article.

POLIOENCEPHALOMALACIA

PEM or cerebrocortical necrosis is a common problem encountered in calves, especially those in feedlots. The disease has been associated with thiamine deficiency, high-sulfur diet, low-roughage diet, high doses of amprolium, cobalt-deficient diet, and molasses-urea diet, as well as ingestion of various toxic plants.[2–4] Although there may not be an exact cause, certainly nutrition plays an important role in the development of the disease. Histologic lesions are primarily necrosis of the gray matter in the brain, similar to lead and/or salt toxicity. In calves, the greatest risk period is between 6 to 18 months of age, with higher susceptibility in younger animals due to lower blood thiamine concentration and intensive feeding systems.[5]

Pathophysiology

Thiamine deficiency has long been recognized for its role in the pathophysiology of PEM in calves. Preruminants depend on ingestion of dietary thiamine, whereas older ruminants rely on rumen bacterial production of thiamine to meet their daily requirement. Thus, when normal rumen production of thiamine is altered or when ingestion is reduced, animals become at risk of deficiency.[3] Brain lesions are thought to be due to impairment of glucose metabolism. Thiamine is known to be necessary in glucose metabolism, playing a role in the Krebs cycle. Insufficient brain glucose will decrease the energy supply to the brain, reducing lipid synthesis, acetylcholine, and other neurotransmitters.[6] Neuronal function will be altered and will eventually lead to clinical signs of PEM.

Bacterial thiaminase has been considered the main factor leading to thiamine deficiency in ruminants with PEM. Thiaminase type I acts by catalyzing the cleavage of thiamine at the methylene bridge between the pyrimidinyl and thiazole ring. Cosubstrate (benzimidazoles, levamisole, or promazine) is required to combine with the pyrimidinyl to form a new compound. Thiaminase type II catalyzes the hydrolysis process between the 2 ring structures of the thiamine molecule. Toxic plants, such as bracken fern (*Pteridium aquilinum*), horsetail (*Equisetum arvense*), and Nardoo fern (*Marsilea drummondii*), contain thiaminase similar to thiaminase type I and have been incriminated in outbreaks of PEM.[4]

Several cases of PEM have been associated with either normal levels of thiamine or treatment failure after thiamine supplementation, therefore other causes were thought to exist than just simple thiamine deficiency. More recently it was discovered that PEM could also be caused by sulfur toxicity. Since the first report of this form of PEM, many cases have been associated with high sulfur in the feed or water.[7–11] The complete pathophysiology has not yet been fully elucidated but was initially thought to be due to inhalation of high quantities of hydrogen sulfide (H_2S) gas eructated by the animal due to the high-sulfur diet.[12] Sulfide is neurotoxic in high concentrations because it inhibits the mitochondrial sulfide oxidation at the level of the cytochrome c oxidase.[13,14] The result is decreased ATP production, leading to decreased energy in the brain.

Recent data by Amat and colleagues[14] have led to a new hypothesis. In this study, cattle were fed either high-sulfur or low-sulfur diets. Thiamine, thiamine monophosphate, and thiamine pyrophosphate were measured in rumen fluid, blood, and brain tissue. No effect of the diet was noticed on ruminal and blood thiamine status but thiamine was increased in the brain of cattle on the high-sulfur diet. Those data were then compared with a group of commercial heifers showing clinical signs of natural PEM. The concentration of thiamine diphosphate was significantly reduced in the brain but free thiamine concentration was increased. The investigators concluded that high dietary sulfur increased metabolic demand for thiamine pyrophosphate and hypothesized that high thiamine demand will eventually lead to thiamine deficiency and cerebrocortical necrosis.

In conclusion, neuronal death, development of malacic lesions, and clinical signs of PEM are due to direct effects of sulfur metabolites on brain tissues and reduction of thiamine in the brain. The interaction between sulfur and thiamine in the development of PEM still needs to be explored further to fully understand the mechanism of sulfur-induced PEM.

Clinical Signs

PEM can present in several different ways, including some animals being found dead without previous clinical signs. Mildly affected animals will appear lethargic, obtunded, and anorectic. Cortical blindness is almost always present and absence of menace response with normal to slow pupillary light reflex is very common. Because of this, the animal will appear disoriented and unaware of its surroundings. Hypersensitivity to sound or touch may also be noticed. The disease often progresses rapidly. The animal will show muscular and head tremors, head-pressing, stargazing, dorsomedial strabismus, and eventually sternal recumbency with muscular incoordination. Eventually, severely affected animals will be in lateral recumbency, comatose, exhibiting severe opisthotonos, and convulsions (leg-paddling movements). Those animals will eventually be found dead. Rectal temperature is usually normal. Video 1 (available online at http://www.vetfood.theclinics.com) shows a 4-month-old Holstein calf that is unable to stand and has cortical blindness, an absent menace response, and exhibits leg-paddling movements. The video also shows marked improvement in the clinical signs approximately 12 to 18 hours after thiamine administration.

Diagnosis

Antemortem diagnosis of PEM is often difficult. Most ruminants with cortical signs are treated with thiamine and response to therapy over 24 hours is used to predict PEM. Rapid improvement in some can be impressive. Cerebrospinal fluid (CSF) collection and analysis has not been shown to be diagnostic. Normal CSF with or without mild mononuclear pleocytosis has been collected from cattle and small ruminants with a PEM diagnosis.[15–17] The main benefit of CSF collection is to allow practitioners to exclude infectious diseases such as listeriosis and bacterial meningitis.

Other antemortem diagnostic tests developed include blood thiamine levels,[18,19] tissue thiamine levels,[20] thiamine pyrophosphate,[21] erythrocyte transketolase activity,[21] erythrocyte concentration of thiamine,[18] rumen thiamine level,[22] and fecal thiaminase activity.[20] Erythrocyte transketolase activity decreases and thiamine pyrophosphate increases with PEM but both measurements are difficult to interpret. Blood thiamine levels typically decrease but are not always reliable. Hill and colleagues[19] proposed a reference range of 75 to 185 nmol/L for cattle and sheep with levels below 50 nmol/L are consistent with deficiency.

In cases of suspected sulfur toxicity, H_2S in rumen fluid and gas, sulfur in blood or tissue, and thiosulfate in the urine can be measured.[9,23] Although concentrations of H_2S in rumen gas and thiosulfate in urine have shown significant increases in cattle with high-sulfur diets, no threshold has been defined yet for PEM. Concentration of H_2S in rumen gas higher than 1000 ppm[24] or 2000 ppm,[12] and of 50 mg/L in urinary thiosulfate, has been associated with consumption of high dietary sulfur when considering diurnal variation associated with feeding schedule.[23] High-sulfur content in water and feed sources should be determined in the case of an outbreak. Maximum tolerable concentration of sulfur for cattle has been established to be 0.40% of the diet for forage-based diet[25] and 0.3% for feedlot animal.[26] Blood lead and sodium concentration can also be measured to exclude those 2 potential differentials.

Necropsy and histopathology will confirm the diagnosis of PEM.[27] Lesions will be localized to the cortex, sometimes extending to the basal and thalamic nuclei, colliculi, and brainstem nuclei. Bilateral and symmetric yellowish discoloration of the gray matter will be observed grossly.[28] The brain will look swollen with flattening and softening of the gyri. Presence of cerebellar or occipital lobe herniation can be present through the foramen magnum and tentorium cerebelli, respectively, with severe brain edema. Histologically, there is diffuse laminar necrosis of the gray matter in the cerebral cortex. Acidophilic neuronal necrosis, intracellular and pericellular edema, gliosis, and neuronophagia can also be noticed. Chronic lesions (2–3 days) will contain blood macrophages. Macroscopic diagnosis can also be confirmed by fluorescence on either fresh or formalin-fixed sections of the brain exposed to Wood lamp (ultraviolet lamp at 365 nm). Necrotic areas will appear bright green as a result of ceroid lipofuscin present in the damaged areas of the brain (**Fig. 1**).

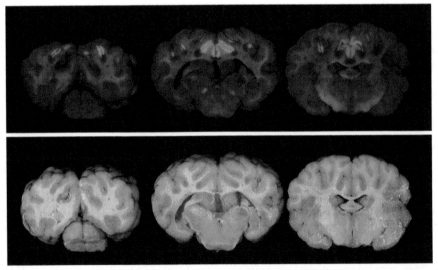

Fig. 1. Coronal sections of the cerebrum from a goat diagnosed with PEM. The top panel shows images of the brain taken under exposure to a Wood lamp. Fluorescent or green areas indicate PEM and result from ceroid lipofuscin present in the necrotic areas of the brain. The bottom panel shows the brain without exposure to the Wood lamp. Small necrotic areas present in the gray matter can be appreciated.

New imaging techniques have shown interesting developments in the last few years. MRI findings of lesions have recently been described in a calf and a goat diagnosed with PEM.[29,30] In both cases, T2-weighted images revealed hyperintense regions along the cerebral cortex confined to the gray matter. The lesions were diffuse, bilateral, and symmetric. No difference in signal intensity between gray and white matter was seen on the T1-weighted images in the calf but the lesion appeared hypointense in the gray matter on the goat MRI. This difference can likely be attributed to the use of a higher quality MRI machine in the second case or may be potentially related to differences in the severity of disease. MRI is able to provide additional information for the clinician as a routine examination; however, its use in bovine practice is certainly limited by cost and availability. MRI will be of greater use in experimental research helping to determine the association between clinical signs and the progression of lesions.

Treatment

Regardless of cause, treatment of PEM primarily involves thiamine supplementation (10–20 mg/kg every q6–8 hours, intravenous [IV], intramuscular [IM], or subcutaneous [SC]).[24] Many investigators have recommended giving the first injection IV, slowly, with subsequent injections given IM or SC to reduce the risk of complications associated with IV thiamine delivery. Improvement should be noticed in the first 24 hours but full recovery can take weeks, depending of the underlying cause. Other treatments should focus on reducing cerebral edema, controlling seizures, and providing supportive care to the animal. Dexamethasone (0.1–0.2 mg/kg, IV or IM), mannitol 20% (1 g/kg, IV) and dimethyl sulfoxide (DMSO) have been used to reduce cerebral edema. Diazepam, phenobarbital, or pentobarbital can be used to control convulsions. Other treatments include limiting access to or removing contaminated water, high-sulfur diet, or toxic plants; parenteral or enteral glucose or glucose precursors for molasses-urea–induced PEM; and antimicrobials to prevent aspiration pneumonia. Practitioners should keep in mind that animals with severe cortical lesions are unlikely to respond to treatment.

Therapeutic interventions in bovine PEM have been recently reviewed.[31] Conclusions of this extensive review were supportive of the use of thiamine in the treatment of bovine PEM. Other treatments, including nonsteroidal anti-inflammatory drugs, dexamethasone, furosemide, and mannitol were either lacking studies to demonstrate efficacy or were not supported by data from the human literature and/or data from induced models of disease. The only other treatment that demonstrated efficacy in laboratory animals was DMSO for treatment of cerebral edema. However, clinical trials have not been done in ruminants and DMSO is prohibited from food animal use in most countries.

Prevention

Prevention of PEM outbreaks should be managed by avoiding access to high sulfur in the feed or water, and supplementing thiamine in the diet (3–10 mg/kg). Frequent analysis of water and feedstuffs to estimate daily sulfur intake would allow rapid correction of the problem. Finally, ruminants should be allowed an adequate period for adaptation to high-concentrate diets. Supplementation with cobalt, copper, zinc, molybdenum, and ferric iron are also helpful.[3,32]

MENINGITIS

Meningitis refers to an inflammation of the meninges and potentially brain. It presents as an occasional sequelae to septicemia, typically in calves less than 30 days of age.

Newborn calves are particularly at risk for developing septicemia because they depend on colostral antibodies and leukocytes (passive transfer of immunity) for immunity. Calves lack a normal adult intestinal flora and, when born in a heavily contaminated environment, colonization of the gastrointestinal tract with virulent bacteria may occur before the establishment of normal flora. Septicemia may also result from bacterial colonization of another site such as the umbilicus. Prognosis in cases of meningitis is often poor; however, treatment may be successful in some cases.

Pathophysiology

Escherichia coli are generally the most common pathogens associated with meningitis in calves; however, other bacteria such as *Salmonella, Campylobacter, Klebsiella*, and different *Staphylococcus* species have been reported.[16,33,34] However, exactly how bacteria get into the meninges is poorly understood. Multiple mechanisms have been proposed, including the development of a sustained and high-grade bacteremia in the highly perfused dural venous system and choroid plexuses, adherence of fimbriae from some strains of *E coli*, and the phagocytosis of the pathogens by circulating monocytes and endocytosis through microvascular endothelial cells.[35] What is apparent is that once bacteria cross into the central nervous system, they are able to survive and proliferate well in the poorly defended CSF. Complement is essentially nonexistent in CSF and there are low numbers of antibodies, leading to inadequate clearance of pathogens from CNS. Gram-negative bacteria also release endotoxins, leading to inflammatory infiltrates that cause thromboses of the arachnoidal or subependymal veins. Congestion or hemorrhagic infarction may follow with subsequent necrosis of nerve cells.

Clinical Signs

Calves with meningitis are typically depressed, lethargic, and have lost their suckle reflex.[33] They often have an extended head and neck and hypopyon (presence of fibrin and white blood cells in the eye) may be seen (**Fig. 2**). Attempts to flex or reposition the neck can result in a tonic extension and thrashing of the limbs. Most cases will present with an elevated rectal temperature unless the calf has already been treated with antiinflammatory drugs. Calves with meningitis almost always have abnormal mentation. As the diseases progresses, profound depression develops and, eventually, the animal becomes comatose and nonresponsive, or may develop seizures.

Diagnosis

Calves with abnormal mentation or with the neurologic signs previously discussed can be strongly suspected of having meningitis. This suspicion is increased further if failure of passive transfer is documented or if a focal infection is present (eg, swollen umbilicus, septic arthritis). However, definitive diagnosis is based on analysis of CSF. Collection of CSF from the lumbosacral space of calves is a fairly simple procedure. Practitioners are encouraged to reference the article by Fecteau and colleagues[35] for pictures of the correct way to position a calf and the proper location to attempt collection of fluid. Typical CSF findings in calves with bacterial meningitis include an increase in both protein and white blood cell concentration, with a dramatic increase in the percentage of nucleated cells that are neutrophils (**Table 1**).[16,33,34] The ratio of CSF to plasma glucose concentration is less than 1 in animals with bacterial meningitis because of bacterial metabolism of glucose in the CSF. Xanthochromia (yellow color) is inconsistent. Free or intracellular bacteria may be observed in some cases. Culture of CSF fluid can be attempted but typically bacterial pathogens are cultured in only 50% to 60% of cases (see **Table 1**).

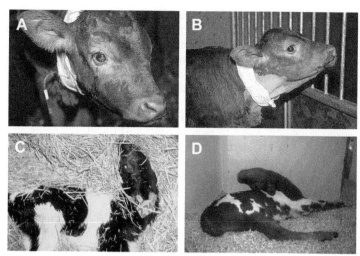

Fig. 2. Calves exhibiting clinical signs of meningitis secondary to septicemia. (*A*) The calf is depressed and maintains an extended neck when manipulated. (*B*) The presence of fibrin and white blood cells in the anterior chamber of the eye (hypopyon) is suspected. (*C, D*) Calves with more advanced meningitis exhibit profound opisthotonus. (*From* Fecteau G, Smith BP, George LW. Septicemia and meningitis in the newborn calf. Vet Clin North Am Food Anim 2009;25:203; with permission.)

Treatment

Overall, the prognosis in cases of bacterial meningitis is very poor. For example, in a case report involving 32 calves, the mortality was 100%.[33] Therefore, humane euthanasia becomes the most appropriate course of action in most cases. In valuable calves, antimicrobial therapy should be based on drugs that can cross the blood-brain barrier and achieve therapeutic concentrations in the CNS. The ratio of a drug in the CSF to blood generally gives a good indication of the potential for that antimicrobial to penetrate the CNS. Because very few of these studies have been conducted in animals, data are, for the most part, extrapolated from human medicine. It is also important to consider the safety margin of drugs. For example, the β-lactams do

Table 1				
Cerebrospinal fluid findings in calves with naturally occurring meningitis				
	Normal	**Meningitis[17]**	**Meningitis[33]**	**Meningitis[16]**
Number of calves	—	11	22	11
Total Protein	<0.4 g/L	3.54 g/L	3.07 g/L	4.14 g/L
Total White Blood Cell Concentration	<10 cells/μl	4365 cells/μL (50–12,600)	4004 cells/μL (130–23,700)	2900 cells/μL (425–30,000)
Lymphocytes (%)	>80–90	6 (0–20)	NR	2 (0–28)
Neutrophils (%)	<10–15	85 (63–100)	73	84 (15–95)
Culture Positive	—	6/9	11/19	3/6

Data represent calves from 3 separate case reports, including mean total protein and total nucleated cell concentrations (with ranges for cell counts when given).
Abbreviation: NR, not reported.

not diffuse very efficiently into the CSF; however, they have a high safety margin and therapeutic concentrations can be achieved in the brain because increased doses can be used without toxicity. In contrast, aminoglycosides diffuse relatively easily across the blood-brain barrier but likely represent a poor choice for meningitis because standard doses are not high enough to achieve therapeutic concentrations in the CSF and higher than standard doses carry a high risk for nephrotoxicity. There is only 1 study that has actually looked at the CSF concentrations of a specific antimicrobial in calves. With labeled doses of florfenicol (20 mg/kg) given IV to calves, the maximum concentration achieved in the CSF was 4.67 plus or minus 1.51 μg/mL at 2 hours after dosing and remained above 1 μg/mL for more than 12 hours.[36] This drug would be quite effective for treating meningitis caused by a pathogen such as *H somnus*, which has a minimal inhibitory concentration (MIC90) for florfenicol of 0.25 μg/mL. However, it would probably not be as effective against *E coli*, which typically has MIC values of at least 8 to 16 μg/mL.

Although broad-spectrum antimicrobials are indicated, *E coli* is the most common isolate from meningitis cases, so it should be the primary target of initial therapy. The choice of antimicrobial for treating meningitis mostly depends on the veterinary drug laws in the country in which the calf is being treated. For example, common recommendations for meningitis treatment in calves have included ceftiofur (5–10 mg/kg q8 hours, IM or IV) or enrofloxacin (5 mg/kg q12 hours, IV).[35] Either of these would likely represent reasonable options; however, both are prohibited in the United States. Labeled doses of ceftiofur (2.2 mg/kg, IM) could be used, or sodium ampicillin (10–20 mg/kg q8h, IV) could possibly be tried. Another potential option is potentiated sulfonamides, such as trimethoprim-sulfamethoxazole dosed at 5 mg/kg (trimethoprim component) every 8 to 12 hours, IV. Potentiated sulfonamides could also be given concurrently with sodium ampicillin or ceftiofur to try and broaden the spectrum of activity. Intrathecal therapy (administering antibiotics directly into the CSF) has not been shown to improve outcome in human medicine and is likely too complicated for use in farm animals.[37] Ancillary therapy with nonsteroidal anti-inflammatory drugs is likely indicated and seizures should be controlled with diazepam (0.1–0.2 mg/kg, IV). Clinical improvement is likely to be slow with duration of therapy likely at least 10 to 14 days, at a minimum.[37]

Prevention

Because meningitis is a sequelae associated with septicemia, prevention is best assured through making sure good colostrum management programs are in place and that calves have adequate ingestion of maternal antibodies. If multiple calves with meningitis are reported from the same herd, environment and farm management practices should also be examined. Outbreaks or clusters of meningitis could be related to specific management problems or risk factors, such as feeding heavily contaminated colostrum, poor umbilical hygiene, overcrowding, or calves being raised in a very dirty environment. Ultimately, meningitis is best controlled by proper management, ensuring good vaccination and colostrum programs, and preventing the occurrence of neonatal septicemia, umbilical infections, and so forth.

HYPERNATREMIA (SODIUM TOXICITY)

Hypernatremia (also known as sodium or salt toxicity) is a relatively common problem encountered in young calves. These cases are generally a result of the calf ingesting excessive concentrations of salt without an adequate balance of water to balance the sodium load. The most common clinical scenarios involve calves ingesting milk replacers that are high in sodium without access to fresh water[38–40] or calves that are being treated for diarrhea that receive oral electrolyte solutions with high sodium concentrations.[41,42] Recently, cases of hypernatremia in calves have been observed associated with the use of high-sodium water on farms. Affected calves are typically less than 3 weeks of age and often (but not always) exhibit neurologic signs.

Pathophysiology

The volume of the extracellular fluid (ECF) is determined by the total body sodium content, whereas the osmolality and sodium concentration of the ECF are determined by sodium and water balance. Multiple control mechanisms work in the body to detect and respond to changes in the osmolality and volume of the ECF. These homeostatic mechanisms primarily control retention and excretion of sodium. Examples of regulatory control include the thirst response (water ingestion) and excretion or retention of sodium by the kidneys. Although it sounds simple, these are under complex control by multiple hormonal pathways, including antidiuretic hormone (ADH), atrial natriuretic peptide (ANP), and the renin-angiotensin-aldosterone system (RAAS), as well as the autonomic nervous system. A complete discussion of the physiology of sodium and water homeostasis is beyond the scope of this article but readers are referred to other recent review articles for more detailed information.[43,44] When calves take in too much sodium, this results in expansion of the ECF at the expense of intracellular fluid to return the osmolality of the blood to normal (relative dehydration). In cases in which there is no water intake, fluid loss is associated with reduction in total body water content (absolute dehydration). In cases of hypernatremia, the brain has to adapt to the hyperosmolar state, which typically involves shrinkage of neurons as water follows concentration gradients and moves into the hyperosmolar CSF and plasma. This results in dehydration of neurons and brain shrinkage. As the brain moves away from the calvaria, disruption of the normal blood supply can occur.[43] High intracellular sodium has also been shown to disrupt neuronal anaerobic glycolysis and normal intracellular ionic gradients.[45] Neurologic signs often worsen during treatment of calves with hypernatremia because rapidly lowering the sodium concentration will allow water to flow into neurons, causing the already shrunken cells to swell, resulting in cerebral edema. This edema can lead to seizures and, in many cases, death.

Clinical Signs

Not all cases of hypernatremia include neurologic signs. Some farms simply report increased calf mortality. Other signs reported include diarrhea, lethargy, depression, and anorexia. Diarrhea has been reported in many calves with sodium toxicity but it is important to recognize that the hypernatremia likely occurred secondary to treatment of the diarrhea. Typical neurologic signs result primarily from cerebral edema and include muscle tremors, ataxia, opisthotonus, and seizures. Video 2 (available online at http://www.vetfood.theclinics.com) shows a 1-week-old Hereford calf with a serum sodium concentration of 187 mEq/L. The calf is exhibiting muscle tremors, head pressing type behavior, and is uncoordinated. Beef cattle have been described as "down and shaking" in the pasture by owners because multiple animals were in lateral recumbency with tremors and seizures after the water supply salt poisoning occurred.[46]

Diagnosis

In animals that are still alive, a routine serum biochemistry panel will provide information on sodium levels. Hypernatremia is defined as a serum or plasma sodium concentration of 160 mEq/L or greater and neurologic signs can be seen. Serum sodium concentrations greater than 180 mEq/L generally indicate a guarded to poor prognosis. Sodium concentrations in the CSF of cattle normally range from 130 to 142 mEq/L in cattle but are typically above 160 mEq/L in animals with hypernatremia.[46] Ocular fluid represents a good sample to submit to the diagnostic laboratory in dead calves because it does not change appreciably with advancing postmortem autolysis and provides a stable representation of sodium levels at the time of death.[47] Ocular fluid sodium concentration is reported to be about 95% of the serum sodium value and levels are significantly elevated in cattle with hypernatremia.[46] In cattle that are dead, the entire brain or cerebral cortex should be submitted to a diagnostic laboratory for sodium analysis and histopathology. Usually, laboratories recommend submitting at least 50 g of fresh brain along with multiple formalin-fixed slices. Typically, there are no gross lesions of the brain apparent at necropsy in cases of hypernatremia and histopathology is nonspecific with cerebral edema present. Therefore, submitting fresh brain and/or ocular fluid for sodium analysis, in addition to requesting histopathology is critical. Sodium concentrations in brain tissue are generally greater than 2000 μg/g (ppm) in calves with hypernatremia.

Treatment

Treatment of calves with chronic hypernatremia is often very difficult and should be reserved primarily for valuable animals. Typical recommendations call for sodium concentrations to be lowered very slowly because replacing free water too rapidly could cause neurons to swell, cerebral edema, and a worsening of neurologic signs. The total body free water deficit can be calculated using the following formula: 0.6 × body weight (kg) × ([current serum sodium concentrations or normal serum sodium concentration] − 1). However, if this fluid is given rapidly, neurologic complications will often arise. In general, the recommendation is to formulate fluids that have a sodium concentration approximately equal to that of the calf.[43,48] This can be done by adding small volumes of hypertonic saline (1.2 mEq/ml) or 23.4% sodium chloride (4 mEq/ml) to whatever fluid type the practitioner has chosen to give the calf. For example, if the calf has an acidemia, additional sodium can be added to isotonic sodium bicarbonate (sodium concentration 156 mEq/L). However, if the calf had a relatively normal pH, additional sodium could be added to 0.9% saline (sodium concentration is 154 mEq/L). The idea is to decrease the sodium level of the calf very slowly over several days to avoid cerebral edema. The following case example illustrates the calculation.

The Hereford calf from Video 2 had a serum sodium concentration of 187 mEq/L. To calculate the free water deficit in this calf, multiply 0.6 × 45 × ([187 − 145] −1) to get a free water deficit of 7.82 L. In this example, 145 was used to represent the normal serum sodium concentration for a calf. If 0.9% saline was given to this calf (154 mEq of sodium per liter), 33 mEq of additional sodium (per liter of fluids) would be needed to reach the calf's serum sodium concentration of 187. The simplest way to do this is to add a small volume of hypertonic saline (33 mEq/1.2 mEq/ml = 27 mL of hypertonic saline added per liter of fluids). Hypertonic saline could be added to isotonic sodium bicarbonate if the calf had an acidemia. Because isotonic sodium bicarbonate has a sodium concentration of 156 mEq/L, 31 mEq of additional sodium would be added. Be careful with adding large volumes of dextrose to these solutions because that will lower the sodium concentration.[43]

Prevention

Hypernatremia is mostly avoidable with proper management. The key becomes preventing either of these from occurring because this condition usually occurs in 1 of the following conditions (1) calf ingests too much sodium without an adequate volume of water in a short period of time or (2) sustained water deprivation. Whole milk is typically fairly low in sodium concentration, averaging about 17 to 28 mmol/L, although this may increase to 35 to 45 mmol/L in late gestation or in cows with mastitis.[49] Therefore, typically, calves fed whole milk have minimal problems with sodium toxicity unless given a large amount of oral electrolytes. Some milk-replacer products can have significantly higher sodium concentrations compared with whole milk. Although there is little published information on the mineral concentration of different milk replacers, sodium concentrations in the 85 to 100 mmol/L range have been measured in milk replacers mixed with distilled water according to label directions. Water quality is another factor that can have a profound effect on the amount of sodium calves ingest. Water that has been through a softening process to remove minerals such as calcium and magnesium often have very high sodium concentrations and, therefore, should not be used to dilute commercial milk replacers unless a water analysis has been performed and sodium levels are less than 100 ppm. In a case report of salt poisoning in calves, milk-replacer samples diluted with farm water had sodium concentrations ranging from 171 to 185 mmol/L.[38] When cases of hypernatremia are diagnosed on a farm, veterinarians should not forget to consider the drinking water source as a possible source of excess sodium.

In addition to watching how much sodium calves are fed in their normal milk diet, attention must also be given to the feeding of oral electrolyte solutions in calves with diarrhea. The optimal concentration of sodium in an oral electrolyte solution is 90 to 130 mmol/L,[50] although some electrolyte products contain levels significantly higher than that when mixed according to label directions.[51] When homemade oral electrolyte products are used or when labeled mixing directions are not followed correctly, sometimes the sodium concentration fed to calves can be extremely high. In some cases, oral electrolyte products are purchased in bulk containers and more powder is added to 2 L of water than indicated in the directions. Multiple case reports describing hypernatremia in calves have involved the feeding of unknown amounts of oral electrolyte solution to calves multiple times per day (Abutarbush and Petrie,[41] 2007; Pringle and Berthiaume,[42] 1988). This situation is exacerbated when calves do not have access to fresh water or when the fresh water also contains high sodium concentrations. In 1 case report, hypernatremia was diagnosed associated with neurologic signs and deaths in a group of 6- to 10-month-old Holstein calves that had access to a salt block without free-choice water available.[52] So, ultimately, paying attention to the calf feeding program and the diarrhea treatment (oral electrolyte) protocol for the farm are critical, along with ensuring calves always have a supply of fresh, good-quality water.

BRAIN ABSCESSES

Abscesses of the nervous system can originate from primary infection in any part of the body that spreads through the circulatory system. Calves often develop abscesses from embolic spread of bacteria from the umbilicus. In addition, brain abscesses can form from the extension of otitis or sinusitis. Clinical signs can vary significantly depending on the region of the brain affected. In cattle, abscesses have been described in basically all parts of the brain, including the cerebrum, cerebellum, and brain stem. *Trueperella pyogenes* is the most frequent cause of brain abscesses in cattle; however, other pathogens have also been described, including *Fusobacterium necrophorum*, *Listeria monocytogenes*, *Bacteroides* species, and *Candida*. Clinical signs are generally slow in onset but progressive as the abscess expands and occupies space in the brain. Forebrain abscesses compress the cerebral

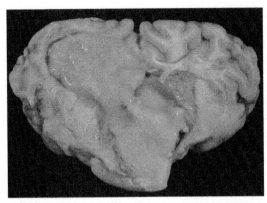

Fig. 3. Brain from the calf shown in Video 3 showing an abscess throughout a significant portion of the cerebrum.

cortex and often cause the functional loss of 1 or both lobes. This often results in blindness of 1 or both eyes. As the abscess gets larger, cortical signs worsen and include propulsive walking, circling, head pressing, head tilt (toward the lesion side), and occasionally unexplained aggression. Video 3 (available online at http://www.vetfood. theclinics.com) shows a 9-month-old Holstein calf that has been exhibiting these clinical signs for approximately 6 months before admission. This calf was humanely euthanized and had a cerebral abscess present at necropsy (**Fig. 3**).

CSF findings in cattle with brain abscesses are variable with some animals being normal (particularly in early cases) and others having very high protein concentrations and marked pleocytosis.[53] Advanced imaging studies, such as computed tomography (CT) or MRI have been shown to be helpful for antemortem diagnosis when they are available (**Fig. 4**).[54] However, definitive diagnosis of brain abscesses are most often

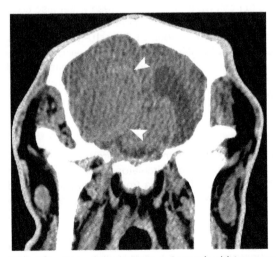

Fig. 4. Transverse CT examination of the brain in a 6-month-old Japanese Black calf with a brain abscess in the right cerebrum. Asymmetric lateral ventricles and the presence of intracranial low absorption masses (*arrowheads*) surrounded by a capsule. The CT values in the lesion were 20 to 30 HU. (*Courtesy of* Dr Kazutaka Yamada of Azabu University, Japan.)

made at necropsy. In general, the neurologic signs are fairly advanced in most cattle with brain abscesses presented to veterinarians and successful treatment has not been described to the authors' knowledge. Treatment with antimicrobials and anti-inflammatory drugs may cause a slight improvement; however, this is usually temporary and the prognosis is almost always grave.

SUPPLEMENTARY DATA

Supplementary data related to this article can be found online at http://dx.doi.org/10.1016/j.cvfa.2016.09.004.

REFERENCES

1. Constable PD. Clinical examination of the ruminant nervous system. Vet Clin North Am Food Anim 2004;20:185–214.
2. Hill FI, Ebbett PC. Polioencephalomalacia in cattle in New Zealand fed chou moellier (Brassica oleracea). N Z Vet J 1997;45:37–9.
3. Cebra CK, Cebra ML. Altered mentation caused by polioencephalomalacia, hypernatremia, and lead poisoning. Vet Clin North Am Food Anim 2004;20:287–302.
4. McKenzie RA, Carmichael AM, Schibrowski ML, et al. Sulfur-associated polioencephalomalacia in cattle grazing plants in the Family Brassicaceae. Aust Vet J 2009;87:27–32.
5. McGuirk SM. Polioencephalomalacia. Vet Clin North Am Food Anim 1987;3:107–17.
6. Amat S, Olkowski AA, Atila M, et al. A review of polioencephalomalacia in ruminants: is the development of malacic lesions associated with excess sulfur intake independent of thiamine deficiency? Vet Med Anim Sci 2013;1:1.
7. Mella CM, Perez-Oliva O, Loew FM. Induction of bovine polioencephalomalacia with feeding system based on molasses and urea. Can J Comp Med 1976;40:104–10.
8. Raisbeck MF. Is polioencephalomalacia associated with high- sulfate diets? J Am Vet Med Assoc 1982;180:1303–5.
9. McAllister MM, Gould DH, Raisbeck MF, et al. Evaluation of ruminal sulfide concentrations and seasonal outbreaks of poliocephalomalacia in beef cattle in a feedlot. J Am Vet Med Assoc 1997;211:1275–9.
10. Niles GA, Morgan SE, Edwards WC. Sulfur-induced polioencephalomalacia in stocker calves. Vet Hum Toxicol 2000;42:290–1.
11. Niles GA, Morgan S, Edwards WC, et al. Effects of dietary sulfur concentrations on the incidence and pathology of polioencephalomalicia in weaned beef calves. Vet Hum Toxicol 2002;44:70–2.
12. Gould DH, Cummings BA, Hamar DW. In vivo indicators of pathologic ruminal sulfide production in steers with diet-induced polioencephalomalacia. J Vet Diagn Invest 1997;9:72–6.
13. Ammann HM. A new look at physiologic respiratory response to H_2S poisoning. J Hazard Mater 1986;13:369–74.
14. Amat S, McKinnon JJ, Olkowski AA, et al. Understanding the role of sulfur-thiamine interaction in the pathogenesis of sulfur-induced polioencephalomalacia in beef cattle. Res Vet Sci 2013;95:1081–7.
15. Little PB, Sorensen DK. Bovine polioencephalomalacia, infectious embolic meningoencephalitis, and acute lead poisoning in feedlot cattle. J Am Vet Med Assoc 1969;155:1892–903.

16. Stokol T, Divers TJ, Arrigan JW, et al. Cerebrospinal fluid findings in cattle with central nervous system disorders: a retrospective study of 102 cases (1990-2008). Vet Clin Pathol 2009;38:103–12.
17. Scott PR. Cerebrospinal fluid collection and analysis in suspected sheep neurological disease. Small Rumin Res 2010;92:96–103.
18. MacPherson A, Moon FE, Voss RC. Biochemical aspects of cobalt deficiency in sheep with special reference to vitamin status and a possible involvement in the aetiology of cerebrocortical necrosis. Br Vet J 1976;132:294–308.
19. Hill JH, Rammell CG, Forbes S. Blood thiamine levels in normal cattle and sheep at pasture. N Z Vet J 1988;36:49–50.
20. Edwin EE, Markson LM, Shreeve J, et al. Diagnostic aspects of cerebrocortical necrosis. Vet Rec 1979;104:4–8.
21. Evans WC, Evans A, Humphreys DJ, et al. Induction of thiamine deficiency in sheep with lesions similar to those of cerebrocortical necrosis. J Comp Pathol 1975;85:253–67.
22. Gabbedy BJ, Richard RB. Polioencephalomalacia of sheep and cattle. Aust Vet J 1977;53:36–8.
23. Drewnoski ME, Ensley SM, Beitz DC, et al. Assessment of ruminal hydrogen sulfide or urine thiosulfate as diagnostic tools for sulfur-induced polioencephalomalacia in cattle. J Vet Diagn Invest 2012;24:702–9.
24. Cebra C, Loneragan GH, Gould DH. Polioencephalomalacia (cerebrocortical necrosis). In: Smith BP, editor. Large animal internal medicine 5th edition. St Louis (MO): Elsevier; 2015. p. 954–6.
25. National Academies of Sciences, Engineering, and Medicine. Nutrient requirements of beef cattle. 8th edition. Washington, DC: National Academy Press; 2016. p. 118–9.
26. Ensley S. Biofuels coproducts tolerance and toxicology for ruminants. Vet Clin North Am Food Anim 2011;27:297–303.
27. Vandevelde M, Higgins R, Oevermann A, editors. Veterinary neuropathology: essentials of theory and practice. Ames(IO): Wiley Blackwell; 2012. p. 108–11.
28. Nietfeld JC. Neuropathology and diagnostics in food animal. Vet Clin North Am Food Anim 2012;28:515–34.
29. Tsuka T, Taura Y, Okamura S, et al. Imaging diagnosis – Polioencephalomalacia in a calf. Vet Radiol Ultrasound 2008;49:149–51.
30. Ertelt K, Oevermann A, Precht C, et al. Magnetic resonance imaging findings in small ruminants with brain disease. Vet Radiol Ultrasound 2016;57:162–9.
31. Apley MD. Consideration of evidence for therapeutic interventions in bovine polioencephalomalacia. Vet Clin North Am Food Anim 2015;31:151–61.
32. Wu H, Meng Q, Yu Z. Evaluation of ferric oxide and ferric citrate for their effects on fermentation, production of sulfide and methane, and abundance of select microbial populations using in vitro rumen cultures. Bioresour Technol 2016;211:603–9.
33. Green SL, Smith LL. Meningitis in neonatal calves: 32 cases (1983-1990). J Am Vet Med Assoc 1992;201:125–8.
34. Scott PR, Penny CD. A field study of meningoencephalitis in calves with particular reference to analysis of cerebrospinal fluid. Vet Rec 1993;133:119–21.
35. Fecteau G, Smith BP, George LW. Septicemia and meningitis in the newborn calf. Vet Clin North Am Food Anim 2009;25:195–208.
36. de Craene BA, Deprez P, D-Haese E, et al. Pharmacokinetics of florfenicol in cerebrospinal fluid and plasma of calves. Antimicrob Agents Chemother 1997;41:1991–5.
37. Philip AG. Neonatal meningitis in the new millennium. Neoreviews 2003;4:e73–80.

38. Ollivett TL, McGuirk SM. Salt poisoning as a cause of morbidity and mortality in neonatal calves. J Vet Intern Med 2013;27:592–5.
39. Pearson EG, Kalifeiz FA. A case of presumptive salt poisoning (water deprivation) in veal calves. Cornell Vet 1982;72:142–9.
40. Rademacher G, Lorenz I. Salt poisoning in calves fed milk replacers as a herd problem. Prakt Tierarzt 1998;79:841–50.
41. Abutarbush SM, Petrie L. Treatment of hypernatremia is neonatal calves with diarrhea. Can Vet J 2007;48:184–7.
42. Pringle JK, Berthiaume LMM. Hypernatremia in calves. J Vet Intern Med 1988;2: 66–70.
43. Angelos SM, Van Metre DC. Treatment of sodium balance disorders. Vet Clin North Am Food Anim 1999;3:587–607.
44. Byers SR, Lear AS, Van Metre DC. Sodium balance and the dysnatremias. Vet Clin North Am Food Anim 2014;30:333–50.
45. Utter MF. Mechanism of inhibition of anaerobic glycolysis of brain by sodium ions. J Biol Chem 1950;185:499–517.
46. Osweiler GD, Carr TF, Sanderson TP, et al. Water deprivation-sodium ion toxicosis in cattle. J Vet Diagn Invest 1995;7:583–5.
47. McLaughlin PS, MaLaughlin BG. Chemical analysis of bovine and porcine vitreous humors: correlation of normal values with serum chemical values and changes with time and temperature. Am J Vet Res 1987;48:467–73.
48. Angelos SM, Smith BP, George LW, et al. Treatment of hypernatremia in an acidotic neonatal calf. J Am Vet Med Assoc 1999;214:1364–7.
49. Gaucheron F. The minerals of milk. Reprod Nutr Dev 2005;45:473–83.
50. Smith GW, Berchtold J. Fluid therapy in calves. Vet Clin North Am Food Anim 2014;30:409–27.
51. Smith GW. Treatment of calf diarrhea: oral fluid therapy. Vet Clin North Am Food Anim 2009;25:55–72.
52. Senturk S, Cihan H. Salt poisoning in beef cattle. Vet Hum Toxicol 2004;46:26–7.
53. Scott PR. Diagnostic techniques and clinicopathologic findings in ruminant neurologic disease. Vet Clin North Am Food Anim 2004;20:215–30.
54. El-Khodery S, Yamada K, Aoki D, et al. Brain abscess in a Japanese Black calf: utility of computed tomography. J Vet Med Sci 2008;70:727–30.

Cerebral Disorders of the Adult Ruminant

John R. Middleton, DVM, PhD

KEYWORDS

- Cerebral disease • Ruminant • Adult

KEY POINTS

- Cerebral disorders are frequently diffuse and can be manifest by alterations in mentation and behavior.
- Clinical signs may include hyperesthesia, obtundation, stupor, head pushing, central blindness, and possibly seizures.
- Many cases are caused by metabolic derangements, toxicity, or infectious agents.
- Because of the limitations of clinical signs and antemortem tests in differentiating cerebral disorders, knowing which diseases can be ruled in or out and how, will help focus disease treatment and control efforts.

INTRODUCTION

Clinical impression suggests that cerebral disorders of the adult ruminant are uncommon in routine practice. Although many diseases can cause cerebral disease in ruminants, many occur in younger animals, and some of these diseases and disorders are reviewed elsewhere in this edition. When cerebral dysfunction is observed in adult ruminants, it is often associated with metabolic derangements such as acid/base and electrolyte imbalance, dehydration, and ketosis.[1]

This article approaches cerebral disorders from the perspective of workup of the adult ruminant with cerebral disease. A discussion of patient history, physical examination findings, differential diagnoses, diagnostic procedures, and general approaches to treatment are presented.

PATIENT HISTORY

Ruminants with cerebral disease generally have a history of altered mentation. Because many of the causes of cerebral disease in ruminants tend to be metabolic, toxic, or infectious, a thorough understanding of the time course of disease onset

Disclosure Statement: The author has nothing to disclose.
Department of Veterinary Medicine and Surgery, College of Veterinary Medicine, University of Missouri, 900 East Campus Drive, Columbia, MO 65211, USA
E-mail address: middletonjr@missouri.edu

Vet Clin Food Anim 33 (2017) 43–57
http://dx.doi.org/10.1016/j.cvfa.2016.09.005
0749-0720/17/© 2016 Elsevier Inc. All rights reserved.

and progression, animal's diet, housing conditions, reproductive status (eg, peripar-turient), stage of production, and recent changes to husbandry are important factors in performing workup on an animal with cerebral disease. Recent changes in behavior should also be noted.

PHYSICAL EXAMINATION

An in-depth discussion of the neurologic examination of the ruminant and neuroana-tomic localization of lesions are reviewed in Gilles Fecteau and colleagues' article, "Neurological Examination of the Ruminant," and Dusty W. Nagy's article, "Diagnostics and Ancillary Tests of Neurologic Dysfunction in the Ruminant," in this issue.

Cerebral or forebrain (cerebral hemispheres, thalamus, and hypothalamus) disease is often caused by metabolic derangement, toxic insult, or an infectious agent; hence, clinical signs are usually diffuse (symmetric) and will include lethargy, obtundation (decreased alertness), dementia (behavioral changes), and head pushing (defined as impedance of forward motion by an immoveable object) with a normal gait when walked on a level surface.[1] With some disorders, excitement and hyperesthesia rather than obtundation may be manifest. Animals with forebrain disease may exhibit central blindness in which the pupillary light response and palpebral reflex are intact, but the menace response is diminished or absent. In contrast to animals with diffuse disease, animals with an asymmetric lesion may circle toward the side of the lesion with propri-oceptive and postural deficits on the side contralateral to the lesion. Contralateral def-icits in proprioception and postural reactions without a head tilt, strabismus, or nystagmus are consistent with a forebrain lesion and differentiate forebrain disease from vestibular disorders. Depending on etiology and severity of the disease, focal or generalized seizures may also be a feature of cerebral disease.

DIFFERENTIAL DIAGNOSES

A multitude of differential diagnoses exists for cerebral or forebrain disease in rumi-nants (**Table 1**). Although the list of differential diagnoses is lengthy, these diseases and disorders seem to be uncommon in adult animals in clinical practice. For the pur-poses of discussion, differential diagnoses are organized according to general cate-gories, including metabolic, infectious, transmissible spongiform encephalopathies (TSEs), parasitic, other, and toxicity/poisoning (see **Table 1**). Toxicoses of the central nervous system are covered in Gene Niles's article, "Toxicoses of the Ruminant Nervous System," in this issue.

Metabolic

Probably the most frequent causes of cerebral clinical signs in the adult ruminant are metabolic disturbances.[1] Alterations in electrolyte concentrations (calcium, magne-sium, sodium, and potassium) and acid/base and hydration status should be evalu-ated in cases presenting with evidence of cerebral or forebrain disease, as these derangements are often associated with lethargy, obtundation, or stupor.

Although hypoglycemia is uncommon in adults, hypoglycemia can result from de-rangements in energy metabolism as seen in ketosis and pregnancy toxemia. In the absence of glucose, the central nervous system becomes dependent on ketones as an energy substrate. Affected animals may exhibit episodic bizarre behavior including hyperesthesia, walking in circles, head pushing, blindness, licking and chewing, and salivation. The nervous system derangement seen in ketosis is thought to be caused

Table 1
Differential diagnoses for adult ruminants with clinical signs of cerebral disease/dysfunction

Disorder/Disease	Animals Affected
Metabolic	
Acid/base imbalance	Bovine, caprine, ovine
Hepatic encephalopathy	Bovine, caprine, ovine
Hypoglycemia	Bovine, caprine, ovine
Hypocalcemia	Bovine, caprine, ovine
Hypomagenesemia	Bovine, ovine
Hypokalemia	Bovine
Ketosis (nervous)/pregnancy toxemia	Bovine, caprine, ovine
Polioencephalomalacia	Bovine, caprine, ovine
Renal encephalopathy	Bovine, caprine, ovine
Infectious	
Bacterial meningitis	Bovine, caprine, ovine
Bovine herpes virus encephalitis	Bovine
Malignant catarrhal fever	Bovine
Pseudorabies	Bovine, caprine, ovine
Rabies	Bovine, caprine, ovine
Sinusitis	Bovine
Small ruminant lentiviruses (CAEV, OPPV)	Caprine, ovine
Sporadic bovine encephalomyelitis (*Chlamydophila pecorum*)	Bovine
West Nile virus	Ovine
TSEs	
BSE	Bovine
CWD	Cervid
Scrapie	Ovine
Parasitic	
Coccidiosis (nervous)	Bovine
C cerebralis	Ovine
P tenuis	Caprine, ovine
Sarcocystis	Bovine
Other	
Foreign animal diseases	
Babesiosis	Bovine
Borna disease	Ovine (bovine, caprine)
Heartwater (*E ruminantium*)	Bovine, caprine, ovine
Louping Ill	Ovine
Theileriosis	Bovine
Trypanosomiasis	Bovine, caprine, ovine
Hydrocephalus	Bovine, caprine, ovine
Idiopathic epilepsy	Bovine, caprine
Space-occupying mass	
Brain abscess	Bovine, caprine, ovine
Brain tumor	
Hematoma	

(*continued on next page*)

Table 1
(continued)

Disorder/Disease	Animals Affected
Trauma	Bovine, caprine, ovine
Toxic	
Ammonia (ammoniated forage)	Bovine
Ethylene glycol	Bovine, caprine, ovine
Grass staggers	Bovine, caprine, ovine
Insecticide	Bovine, caprine, ovine
Lead	Bovine, caprine, ovine
Nitrofurazone	Bovine, caprine, ovine
Organochlorine	Bovine, caprine, ovine
Propylene glycol	Bovine, caprine, ovine
Plants	Bovine, caprine, ovine
Salt (Sodium)	Bovine, caprine, ovine
Urea	Bovine

Note: Toxicoses are listed as differentials but not discussed in this article (See Gene Niles's article, "Toxicoses of the Ruminant Nervous System," in this issue).

Adapted from Van Metre DC, Mackay RJ. Localization and differentiation of neurologic diseases. In: Smith BP, editor. Large animal internal medicine. 5th edition. St Louis (MO): Elsevier Mosby; 2015; and Constable PD. Ruminant neurologic diseases. Vet Clin North Am Food Anim Pract 2004; xi–xii.

by the conversion of acetoacetic acid to isopropyl alcohol in the rumen, acidosis, or the lack of glucose to support normal nervous tissue function.

Polioencephalomalacia is a description of the necrosis (malacia) seen histologically in the gray (polio) matter of the brain (encephalon). The necrosis results from alterations in cellular metabolism leading to decreased production of adenosine triphosphate, which ultimately leads to cellular necrosis. Several potential inciting causes include thiamine deficiency, sulfur toxicity, and lead toxicity. Sodium toxicity with or without water deprivation can also cause polioencephalomalacia, but the cellular necrosis occurs due an osmotic gradient caused by an accumulation of intracellular sodium in brain cells that pulls free water intracellularly, causing cell rupture when the animal senses thirst and rehydrates. Polioencephalomalacia is reported to occur in animals from a few weeks to several years of age.[2] A variety of clinical signs are seen. In the subacute form, a rapid onset of clinical signs includes staggering that progresses to bilateral blindness, dorsomedial strabismus, head pushing, and bruxism.[3] In the acute form, animals are found recumbent and comatose and may exhibit seizures[3] (See Vincent Dore and Geof Smith's article, "Cerebral Disorders of Calves," in this issue, for a more detailed synopsis on polioencephalomalacia).

Hepatic encephalopathy has been reported in goats, sheep, and cattle.[4–6] The underlying mechanisms for the encephalopathy are poorly understood, and several factors may be at play including hypoglycemia, hyperammonemia, and toxic compounds escaping hepatobiliary degradation and excretion. Although congenital defects causing portosystemic shunting seem to be the major cause of hepatic encephalopathy in young animals,[4,6] hepatic lipidosis[7] and toxic insults to the liver (eg, plant toxicity or mycotoxins) seem to be the cause in adults.

Renal (uremic) encephalopathy was reported in 2 cows[8,9] and a goat.[10] In 2 of the cases (1 cow and 1 goat), no antemortem clinical findings were reported.[8,10]

The 5-year-old cow reported on by Dunigan and colleagues[9] was presented for weight loss and ataxia of 1 week's duration. At the time of presentation, the cow was anxious, disoriented, ataxic, blind, hypermetric in the forelimbs, and 8% dehydrated. Biochemical abnormalities included severe azotemia, hypomagnesemia, hypocalcemia, hypokalemia, hypochloremia, hyperphosphatemia, hypoalbuminemia, and hyperglycemia. Urinalysis found isosthenuria, proteinuria, and glucosuria. Despite fluid therapy the azotemia persisted, and the cow was euthanized. Although renal lesions consistent with a toxic insult were detected histologically, no histologic changes were seen in the central nervous tissues. The authors concluded that the neurologic signs were likely caused by the renal failure. In both the goat and cow that received the postmortem diagnosis, a spongiform encephalomyelopathy attributed to the renal disease was reported.[8,10] The cause of the encephalopathy is thought to be related to increased concentrations of organic acids or phosphorous, imbalances in amino acid concentrations, changes in calcium concentrations, changes in parathyroid hormone activity, or altered neurotransmitter activity.[9]

Infectious

Infectious causes of cerebral disease are generally infrequent in adult ruminants. Although bacterial meningitis can occur in adults, it is more commonly seen in younger animals.[11,12] *Histophilus somni* can cause meningitis in cattle but usually in juvenile cattle in feedlots.[12] Listeriosis can also be associated with meningitis in adult ruminants, but this organism tends to have a tropism for the brainstem and spinal cord rather than the cerebrum. Bacterial meningitis secondary to extension of a frontal sinusitis is also possible. Sporadic bovine encephalitis caused by *Chlamydophila pecorum*, an obligate intracellular gram-negative bacteria, causes rare outbreaks of disease with mortality reportedly highest in calves.[13] The organism causes multisystemic disease including fever, respiratory disease, enteritis, and stiffness. A meningoencephalitis develops, which leads to progression of clinical signs and death within 4 to 10 days.[13]

Viral causes of cerebral dysfunction include bovine herpes virus encephalitis (BHV-1 and BHV-5), malignant catarrhal fever caused by ovine herpes virus 2 (sheep associated; worldwide) or alcelaphine virus 1 (wildebeest associated; Africa), pseudorabies, rabies, small ruminant lentiviruses (maedi-Visna or ovine progressive pneumonia [OPPV], and caprine arthritis encephalitis virus [CAEV]), and West Nile virus. Bovine herpes virus encephalitis is uncommon and usually occurs in calves less than 6 weeks of age; however, a recent case report suggests disease can occur in adult cattle.[14] The head and eye form of malignant catarrhal fever can include cerebral signs of dementia, head pushing, and, terminally, convulsions, but similar to BHV-1 and BHV-5 encephalitis, malignant catarrhal fever–associated encephalitis is rare in clinical practice in North America.

Pseudorabies is caused by suid herpesvirus 1 and is manifest by an acute encephalitis that is frequently fatal in ruminants. Swine are the natural hosts for pseudorabies, and although the virus can infect a multitude of mammals including cattle, sheep, and goats, disease in these animals is rare. Outbreaks have been reported in which ruminants are housed in close proximity to swine. Pseudorabies was eradicated from domestic swine in the United States in 2004,[15] but feral swine present a potential reservoir for infection of domesticated livestock. Rabies is caused by a rhabdovirus that can infect most mammals usually via a bite wound. Occurrence is worldwide with the exception of a few island nations that have managed to remain rabies free. Infected wildlife hosts (eg, bat, skunk, raccoon, fox, and coyote) are the reservoir for the virus, and the virus usually dead ends in nonreservoir hosts. A variety of clinical manifestations can occur including a hyperexcitable state referred to as *furious rabies* and a depressed state referred to as *dumb rabies*.[16] The dumb form is most prevalent in cattle.[16] Both pseudorabies and rabies are reportable diseases.

In small ruminants, lentivirus infections can manifest as cerebral disease. Neurologic signs are rare with OPPV in sheep. In goats, CAEV can cause a leukoencephalomyelitis usually in animals younger than 1 year. West Nile virus encephalitis (an arthropod-borne single-stranded enveloped RNA virus transmitted by mosquitoes of the genus *Culex*) is more commonly reported in horses, but has been reported in isolated cases in sheep in North America and Europe.[17,18]

Transmissible Spongiform Encephalopathies

TSEs have been reported in numerous mammalian species, including sheep and goats (scrapie), cattle (bovine spongiform encephalopathy [BSE]), cervidae (chronic wasting disease), mink (transmissible mink encephalopathy), cats (feline spongiform encephalopathy), and human beings (kuru, Creutzfeldt Jakob disease, and others).[19] These diseases share features including a prolonged latent period, a uniformly progressive and eventually fatal clinical course, and clinical signs, which include weight loss and deteriorating neurologic function, the absence of a host immune response to infection, and characteristic histologic signs.[19] Histologically, there is an accumulation of proteinaceous plaques within the nervous system.[20,21] The proteinaceous plaques are made up of a host protein, called a *prion* (PrP), the structure of which has been altered, making it resistant to normal host catabolic processes (PrP^{res}). The infectious agent thus seems to be a self-replicating abnormal protein. Disease can be a spontaneous event, can occur by facilitated transmission by feeding animal protein containing the abnormal prion (eg, BSE), or by vertical transmission (eg, scrapie).[19] In many cases a genetic susceptibility to accumulation of the abnormal prion is suspected. Transmissible spongiform encephalopathies were extensively reviewed in the previous edition on ruminant neurologic diseases.[19] In this article, BSE, scrapie, and chronic wasting disease (CWD) are briefly reviewed and updates provided where possible.

Bovine spongiform encephalopathy

BSE is a subacute TSE of cattle that was first recognized in the United Kingdom in November 1986; however, examination of archived tissues suggested that cattle had the disease in April 1985.[22] Bovine spongiform encephalopathy cases quickly became recognized throughout the United Kingdom and Ireland, and BSE is now recorded in 27 countries around the world including countries in Europe and the Middle East, Japan, Canada, Brazil, and the United States.[23] Additionally, BSE has been documented in imported cattle in Oman and the Falkland Islands.[23] In North America, surveillance programs have identified 21 cases (20 native-born cattle and 1 cow imported from the United Kingdom) of BSE in Canada and 3 cases in native-born cattle in the United States (Texas, 2005; Alabama, 2006; California, 2012).[23]

Although the true origins of BSE are unknown, experts agree that BSE is caused by the conversion of the normal cellular prion protein (PrP^c) to its abnormal form (PrP^{res}).[24–26] The consensus is that the infectious agent is the self-replicating abnormal prion protein. The BSE outbreak in the United Kingdom, which peaked in 1992, has been linked to feeding contaminated ruminant-origin meat and bone meal (MBM) to cattle.[24,25] Investigations into the origin of BSE were not conclusive as to the source of the abnormal prion in the MBM, but several risk factors were elucidated, including alterations in UK rendering practices in the early 1980s.[26] One hypothesis was that BSE may have arisen from scrapie because of the high ratio of sheep to cattle in the United Kingdom, with about 5,000 to 10,000 cases per year of scrapie occurring at the time, which would have meant a high concentration of scrapie-infected material in MBM.[24] An alternative hypothesis put forth in the BSE Inquiry by Phillips and colleagues[25] was that the BSE agent was not derived from scrapie, but was a novel TSE that arose in cattle in the 1970s and was recycled and amplified by feeding MBM containing infected tissues from affected cattle back to cattle. Although horizontal and vertical transmission are thought to occur with scrapie,[27] these methods of disease transmission seem to play an insignificant role with BSE. Genetic susceptibility to the disease has been suggested because offspring of BSE affected dams are 3.2 times more likely to get the disease.[28–30]

Advances in the understanding of BSE led to the identification of different types of BSE based on characteristics of the abnormal prion. Using western blot, BSE can now be differentiated into 3 types: classical (C type), L type, and H type. The so-called, atypical L type and H type derive their names from the mass (L = Low; H = High) of the unglycosylated isoform of the PrP^{res} protein. The 3 cases of BSE identified in native-born US cattle have been characterized as atypical (L type or H type) by western blot, suggesting they were spontaneous occurrences not related to cattle feeding practices. These atypical types have also been found in cases of BSE in Europe in cattle born after the ban on feeding ruminant-derived protein to livestock.[31]

Studies regarding the pathogenesis of BSE have largely relied on measuring the infectivity of tissues from affected cattle using bioassays in mice, sheep, or cattle. Experimental challenge studies showed infectivity in brain, spinal cord, dorsal root ganglia, trigeminal ganglion, distal ileum, and palatine tonsil with timing of infectivity after experimental exposure ranging from 6 to 40 months depending on tissue examined.[32] In naturally occurring clinical disease, infectivity is detected in the brain, spinal cord, and dorsal root ganglia but not the retropharyngeal, mesenteric, and popliteal lymph nodes. From these studies, the mean incubation period is estimated to be around 45 months (range, 33–55 months).[32]

Unlike other TSEs, BSE was found to cross species barriers. Bovine spongiform encephalopathy has been implicated as the cause of new variant of Creutzfeldt-Jakob disease in humans, feline spongiform encephalopathy in zoo and domestic felidae, and several cases of spongiform encephalopathy in exotic ruminants in zoologic parks in the United Kingdom.[19] Ingestion of ruminant-derived protein has been implicated in each instance. Because of the zoonotic potential of BSE, and based on the infectivity data described above, a list of Specified Risk Materials (tissues that have the potential to transmit the disease to humans through ingestion) was developed, and, in some countries, regulations limiting the age (<30 months in the United Kingdom) at which cattle can be slaughtered for human consumption have been implemented.

Disease manifestation in cattle coincides with pathogenic changes occurring in the brain tissue. The neuropathology is characterized by the presence of vacuolation of brainstem gray matter resulting from neuronal cell death.[22] There is an accumulation of PrP^{res} in brain tissue, which is sometimes associated with the formation of amyloid plaques.[33] The exact mechanism by which neuronal cell death occurs is not fully understood, but it has been proposed that the abnormal prion is neurotoxic through a variety of mechanisms that have not been fully characterized.[33]

Disease incubation ranges from 2 to 8 years with reported age of onset of clinical disease ranging from 22 months to 15 years.[26,34] The disease tends to be slowly progressive, resulting in death 2 weeks to 6 months after initial signs. Clinical signs may wax and wane and include apprehensiveness, nervousness, hyperesthesia, reluctance to negotiate obstacles, reluctance to be milked, aggression toward humans and other animals, manic kicking during milking, head shyness and low head carriage, hypermetria, tremors, ataxia, and progressive loss of body condition and milk yield.[35] According to Saegerman and colleagues,[36] the most frequent clinical profile for a cow with BSE is apprehension or nervousness combined with hyperesthesia and ataxia observed over a 15-day period. A small proportion of animals may show true "mad cow" syndrome manifest by aggression and manic behavior.

BSE is a reportable disease with no definitive antemortem diagnostic tests. Diagnosis is made postmortem by histologic examination of the brainstem or immunodetection of PrP[res] in brainstem by immunohistochemistry, immunoblotting, or an enzyme-linked immunosorbent assay. Histologically, lesions are characterized by bilaterally symmetric intracytoplasmic vacuolation of brainstem gray matter and neurons.

The disease is not treatable. Disease prevention is centered on national and regional control and surveillance programs. By banning the practice of feeding ruminant-derived MBM to livestock, the United Kingdom was able to eventually control the outbreak of what is now termed *classical BSE*. In the United Kingdom, no cases of BSE have been reported in 2016 (data as of April) with less than 10 cases being reported annually for the last 5 years.[23]

Scrapie

Scrapie, the oldest known TSE, is believed to have entered the North American sheep population through importation of infected sheep from the United Kingdom early in the 20th century.[37] Many countries, including the United States, are endemically infected with scrapie.

Like most TSEs, scrapie has a prolonged latent period with peak incidence of clinical disease occurring between 2 and 5 years of age. Horizontal and vertical transmission are reported with scrapie; hence, the prolonged latent period is critically important because ewe's infected with scrapie will have ample opportunity to transmit the disease to their offspring, and lambs born to other ewes before they themselves manifest with clinical disease.[27,38,39] Numbers of animals in a flock showing clinical signs at any given time is, thus, also low because of the prolonged and varied incubation period.

Resistance to scrapie is linked to polymorphisms at codons A136V, R154H, and R171Q of the prion protein gene.[40] Although the ARR allele has been associated with resistance to scrapie, scrapie is still detected in some sheep that are ARR homozygous.[40] The AHQ, ARH, ARQ, and VRQ alleles are generally associated with susceptibility to scrapie. Hence, breeding programs can be designed to select for animals with an ARR allele. One review suggested that such selection has not been shown to have a negative impact on production parameters, but there was a paucity of data relating PrP genotype to disease traits.[40]

Clinically, scrapie is a slowly progressive debilitating disease with progression taking from 2 months to as long as a year. Clinical course in goats seems to be shorter and rarely exceeds 6 months.[19] Early clinical signs may be unapparent. With progression, clinical signs include severe weight loss, poor appetite, pruritis and wool loss, and neurologic signs.[19] Neurologic signs can include altered mentation, hyperesthesia, head bob, muscle fasciculations, hypermetria, dysphonia, dysphagia, blindness, and uncoordinated muscular movements.[19] Early evidence of the altered mental state may include self-imposed isolation from the flock or apparent aggression directed at handlers, other sheep, herding dogs, or inanimate objects. As clinical signs become more severe, the degree of depression increases, affected sheep may become recumbent, and in the latter stages sheep may have seizures. The classic and most useful clinical sign is the response to scratching or light pressure over the withers, which will cause sheep to raise their head, point their muzzle dorsally, elevate their upper lip, lick their lips, and make chewing movements. Although none of these clinical signs are pathognomonic, close questioning of the client usually reveals a protracted, progressive clinical course, effectively ruling out most other causes of neurologic disease in sheep.

As with BSE, scrapie is a reportable and regulated disease, and control of the disease falls within the scope of government control and surveillance programs. There is no effective treatment. Definitive diagnosis is made by postmortem examination of brain tissues or antemortem/postmortem testing of lymphoid tissue (third eyelid, rectoanal lymphoid tissue, tonsil, or retropharyngeal lymph node).[41] Approved diagnostic tests include enzyme-linked immunosorbent assay, western blot, and immunohistochemistry.[41] Once diagnosed, regulatory authorities will determine the fate of the affected animal(s) and rest of the flock. Because of the potential for vertical transmission in utero, retaining lambs from ewes identified as scrapie positive is not recommended. Selection of scrapie-resistant sheep flocks can be achieved through genetic testing of resistant PrP genotypes (see earlier discussion) and evaluating pedigrees for familial evidence of the disease.

Chronic wasting disease
CWD is a TSE of deer and elk that was first reported in 1967 in northern Colorado and southeastern Wyoming; its origin is unknown.[42] CWD is documented in farmed and free-ranging deer and elk in 2 Canadian provinces (Alberta and Saskatchewan), 22 US states (Colorado, Illinois, Iowa, Kansas, Maryland, Michigan, Minnesota, Missouri, Montana [captive facility; depopulated], Nebraska, New Mexico, New York, North Dakota, Oklahoma [captive facility; depopulated], Pennsylvania, South Dakota, Texas, Utah, Virginia, West Virginia, Wisconsin, and Wyoming) and in the Republic of Korea.[43,44] Clinical signs include chronic weight loss, behavioral changes, and neurologic signs. The incubation period of the disease ranges from 18 months to 3 years. Both vertical and horizontal transmission can occur in cervids; however, transmission between cervids and domestic livestock or humans is currently not thought to occur.[19] The United States Geological Survey, National Wildlife Health Center has ongoing research to (1) understand disease transmission, patterns of infection, and infection rates based on gender and age of the animal; (2) indicate genetic resistance to CWD and tools for understanding CWD epidemics; (3) understand the role infected deer carcasses play in disease transmission and how feeding and baiting may influence transmission patterns; and (4) explore the susceptibility of small mammals and their potential role in CWD transmission.[44] As with other TSEs, CWD is a reportable disease that is not treatable and usually fatal.

Parasitic

Parasitic infections that can have cerebral disease manifestations include coccidiosis, *Coenurus cerebralis*, *Sarcocystis*, and aberrant parasite migration (eg, *Parelaphostrongylus tenuis*).

Coccidiosis
Nervous coccidiosis is a neurologic manifestation of an enteric infection with *Eimeria* spp. in cattle, sheep, and goats. The disease is usually seen in young stock, particularly animals on feed, and the neurologic syndrome is thought to be caused by a heat-labile neurotoxin produced by the parasite.[45,46] Clinical signs are often preceded by an episode of bloody diarrhea. Nervous system signs may include depression, incoordination, twitching, and hyperesthesia followed by recumbency, opisthotonus, tremors, horizontal nystagmus, frothing at the mouth, vocalization, muscle fasciculations, and seizures. Prognosis is poor, and death usually occurs 1 to 5 days after the onset of clinical signs.[45]

Coenurus cerebralis

C cerebralis is the intermediate stage of the life cycle of the canine tapeworm, *Taenia multiceps*.[45] The canid hosts shed eggs in their feces, which are ingested by grazing ruminants. The ingested eggs hatch into larvae in the small intestine, enter the bloodstream, and travel to the central nervous system (CNS) where they mature into *C cerebralis*. When the ruminant dies and its brain is ingested by a carnivore, the life cycle is completed. Clinical signs can result from the larval migration through the CNS or from a space-occupying lesion effect.[45]

Sarcocystis

Several species of *Sarcocystis* infect the CNS of ruminants, each with a nonruminant definitive host.[45] The definitive host sheds sporocysts on the pasture, which are ingested by ruminants, hatch in the small intestine, and enter mesenteric arteries where they become sporozoites in endothelial cells. Eventually, merozoites enter other tissues, including the muscle and CNS, and encyst as sarcocysts. When the ruminant dies and its tissues are ingested by the definitive host, the life cycle is completed. Ruminants are generally immune and do not show clinical signs. In nonimmune ruminants, clinical signs may range from fever, anorexia, and weight loss to ataxia or cerebral clinical signs. Although infection is common, clinical CNS disease is rare.[45]

Parelaphostrongylus tenuis

P tenuis, referred to as the *meningeal worm*, is a parasite of white-tail deer whose intermediate host is the snail.[46] The adult parasite inhabits the meninges of the brain of the white-tail deer and is generally nonpathogenic in its definitive host. Eggs from the adult parasite enter the venous circulation, travel to the lungs, and are then coughed up, swallowed, and shed in feces. Larvae are ingested by snails and undergo development from L1 to L3. When the snail is ingested, larvae are released into the gastrointestinal tract and migrate to the spinal cord. In the white-tail, the adult then develops in the meninges (prepatent period approximately 80–90 d); however, in the aberrant host, the migrating larvae damage the spinal cord and brain causing a severe inflammatory response. Clinical signs often include spinal ataxia. Forebrain disease, although possible, is not often seen in clinical cases. Although the disease is often associated with New World camelids, sheep and goats can be affected.

Foreign Animal Diseases

Several diseases termed *exotic* or *foreign animal diseases* have the potential to cause cerebral clinic signs including babesia, borna disease, heartwater (*Ehrlichia ruminantium*), louping ill, theileriosis, and trypanosomiasis.[45,47]

Babesiosis is a tick-borne protozoal disease of ruminants transmitted by ticks of the *Boophilus* genus.[45] Infections in ruminants result in intravascular and extravascular hemolysis and renal and liver failure. On occasion an acute encephalitis may occur with clinical signs including fever, decreased feed intake, and evidence of cortical disease.

Borna disease is a viral encephalitis that can affect multiple mammalian species including ruminants.[45,47] It is suspected that small mammals such as bats and voles serve as a reservoir, and the virus is transmitted by contact with nasal and lacrimal secretions. The disease seems to be localized to central Europe in the upper Rhine valley.

Heartwater (*E ruminantium*) is a rickettsial disease transmitted by ticks of the *Amblyomma* genus.[45,47] The disease occurs in sub-Saharan Africa and the West Indies. Clinical signs can include fever, decreased feed intake, respiratory distress, cyanosis, and CNS signs associated with forebrain dysfunction. Mortality rate is variable in sheep and cattle, but may reach 90% in Angora goats.[45] Animals that recover or live in endemic areas develop immunity; however, Angora goats seem to be the exception and are highly susceptible to the disease.

Louping ill is a tick-borne viral encephalitis primarily of sheep that has been reported in various parts of Europe.[45,47] Disease can occur in humans, horses, and other ruminant species. Outbreaks seem to prevail in wet, swampy areas. Clinical signs include fever, decreased feed intake, and CNS signs including a characteristic bunny-hop gait. As the disease progresses, clinical signs of forebrain disease become manifest. The etiologic agent can be shed in milk presenting a potential zoonosis when unpasteurized dairy products are consumed.

Theileria annulata and *Theileria parva* are capable of causing cerebral disease in cattle.[45,47] Although both *Bos taurus* and *Bos indicus* breeds are susceptible, disease severity is greater in *B taurus* breeds.[45] Clinical signs can include fever, lymphadenopathy, nasal and ocular discharge, tachycardia, facial edema, gangrenous dermatitis, dyspnea, mucous membrane pallor, and neurologic deficits.[45] Animals that recover are persistently infected.

Trypanosomiasis[45,47] is a protozoal infection of African cattle that is transmitted by the tsetse fly. Infection results in fever, anemia, icterus, petechial hemorrhage, melena, and epistaxis. Clinical signs of the encephalitic form include depression, ataxia, proprioceptive deficits, knuckling, head pushing, circling, and ultimately coma and seizures a few days before death.[45]

Miscellaneous

Normotensive hydrocephalus (hydranencephaly) is associated with fetal infection by several viruses including aino, akabane, bluetongue, border disease, bovine viral diarrhea virus, Cache Valley, and Schmallenberg virus; thus, CNS clinical signs are usually manifest at a young age.[45] Hypertensive hydrocephalus, however, can occur in adult ruminants associated with an acquired obstruction of the ventricular system, for example, parasite migration, neoplastic mass, abscess, or meningitis.[45]

Space-occupying lesions can include abscesses (pituitary or brain), hematoma, and neoplasia. Although *Trueperella pyogenes* is most frequently isolated organism from pituitary or brain abscesses in ruminants, several other bacterial pathogens have been isolated.[45] Several different tumors have been documented in the CNS of ruminants, both primary and secondary (metastatic).[48] Lymphosarcoma seems to be the most frequent metastatic brain tumor.[48] Clinical signs of space-occupying masses depend on size and location within the CNS.

Although epilepsy is rare in ruminants, it can occur and may be secondary to an acquired disease or disorder or be primary (idiopathic). Cases of idiopathic epilepsy may have a genetic predilection, and familial epilepsy has been described in cattle.[49]

Trauma to the head may lead to impingement of skeletal structures on the cerebrum. Additionally, swelling, edema, or hemorrhage caused by the traumatic event may compress cerebral tissues leading to clinical signs. A head injury may not be overtly obvious, and concomitant clinical signs such as epistaxis or peripheral swelling may aid in making a diagnosis when the event was not observed.

DIAGNOSTICS

Diagnostic and ancillary tests for neurologic dysfunction in ruminants are discussed in detail in Dusty W. Nagy's article, "Diagnostics and Ancillary Tests of Neurologic Dysfunction in the Ruminant," in this issue. Briefly, antemortem ancillary tests that are commonly used to assist in differentiating cerebral disorders include cerebrospinal fluid collection with cytology and fluid analysis, serology, virus isolation, culture, or polymerase chain reaction for infectious etiologies. Less common would be imaging modalities such as radiography, computed tomography, and MRI. The latter usually require a referral facility.

Cerebrospinal fluid (CSF) can be easily collected from the lumbosacral region with a minimum of expertise and equipment with the animal awake or sedated, and although a definitive diagnosis can infrequently be made on CSF fluid analysis and cytology alone, this test can help rule in or out certain diseases. For example, an eosinophilc pleocytosis may indicate an aberrant parasite migration, whereas a mononuclear pleocytosis may indicate listeriosis, polioencephalomalacia, or viral encephalitis. Serology for lentiviruses help rule in the agent as a potential cause but will not confirm the diagnosis, as many animals can be infected but not have central nervous system manifestations. Virus isolation, bacterial/fungal culture or polymerase chain reaction, either on CSF or in some cases peripheral blood, can help focus the diagnosis on infectious etiologies. In many cases, a definitive diagnosis can only be made postmortem after histologic examination or specialized diagnostic (eg, immunodiagnostics) testing of brain tissue.

TREATMENT

Etiology-specific treatments for cerebral disorders are beyond the scope of this article. Generally speaking, the clinical signs associated with the aforementioned diseases and disorders occur because of a neurodegenerative process or because of swelling, edema, or metabolic derangements. As discussed above, many cases of cerebral dysfunction in adult ruminants may be metabolic in origin. Hence, correction of fluid deficits and acid/base and electrolyte imbalances will be an important component of therapy. With specific metabolic disorders such as polioencephalomalacia, thiamine may be indicated. Reducing swelling and edema by use of an anti-inflammatory or diuretic may also be warranted. For infectious etiologies such as bacterial meningitis or listeriosis, parenteral antibiotics such as oxytetracycline or penicillin will be an important component of the overall therapeutic regimen. Some diseases, as illustrated above, are not treatable (eg, BSE, scrapie, CWD, rabies), and several of the diseases discussed have regulatory or public health implications.

SUMMARY

Although clinical impression suggests that cerebral disorders of adult ruminants are not common, an understanding of the common differential diagnoses is important to protecting animal and human health. When cerebral disorders are noted in adult ruminants, the most common causes are likely metabolic, toxic, or infectious. Many of the diseases discussed above cannot be easily differentiated from one another based on clinical signs or antemortem diagnostic tests alone. Knowing which diseases can be ruled in or out and how will help the practitioner make case management decisions and have broader impact through recognizing index cases of emergent diseases, reducing exposure to zoonotic pathogens (eg, rabies, listeria, BSE), and mitigating disease outbreaks.

REFERENCES

1. Constable PD. Clinical examination of the ruminant nervous system. Vet Clin North Am Food Anim Pract 2004;20:197, 210–11.

2. Gabbedy BJ, Richards RB. Polioencephalomalacia of sheep and cattle. Aust Vet J 1977;53:36–8.

3. Cebra CK, Cebra ML. Altered mentation caused by polioencephalomalacia, hypernatremia, and lead poisoning. Vet Clin North Am Food Anim Pract 2004;20: 287–302.

4. Kinde H, Pesavento PA, Loretti AP, et al. Congenital portosystemic shunts and hepatic encephalopathy in goat kids in California: 11 cases (1999-2012). J Vet Diagn Invest 2014;26:173–7.

5. Sargison ND, Scott PR, Wislon DJ, et al. Hepatic encephalopathy associated with cobalt deficiency and white liver disease in lambs. Vet Rec 2001;149:770–2.

6. Marcal VC, Oevermann A, Bley T, et al. Hepatic encephalomyelopathy in a calf with congenital portosystemic shunt (CPSS). J Vet Sci 2008;9:807–11.

7. Bobe G, Young JW, Beltz DC. Invited review: pathology, etiology, prevention, and treatment of fatty liver in dairy cows. J Dairy Sci 2004;87:3105–24.

8. Summers BA, Smith CA. Renal encephalopathy in a cow. Cornell Vet 1985;75: 524–30.

9. Dunigan C, Tyler J, Valdez R, et al. Apparent renal encephalopathy in a cow. J Vet Intern Med 1996;10:39–41.

10. Radi ZA, Thomsen BV, Summers BA. Renal (uremic) encephalopathy in a goat. J Vet Med A Physiol Clin Med 2005;52:397–400.

11. Green SL, Smith LL. Meningitis in neonatal calves: 32 cases (1983-1990). J Am Vet Med Assoc 1992;201:125–8.

12. Fecteau G, George LW. Bacterial meningitis and encephalitis in ruminants. Vet Clin North Am Food Anim Pract 2004;20:363–77.

13. Mohamad KY, Rodolakis A. Recent advances in the understanding of *Chlamydophila pecorum* infections, sixteen years after it was named as the fourth species of the Chlamydiaceae family. Vet Res 2010;41:27.

14. Rissi DR, Barros CS. Necrotizing meningoencephalitis in a cow. Vet Pathol 2013; 50:926–9.

15. Pseudorabies (Aujeszky's Disease) and its eradication: A review of the U.S. Experience. United States Department of Agriculture, Animal and Plant Health Inspection Service. Technical Bulletin No. 1923.

16. Berthelin CF, George LW. Rabies. In: Smith BP, editor. Large animal internal medicine. 5th edition. St Louis (MO): Elsevier Mosby; 2015. p. 943–5.

17. Kecskemeti S, Bajmocy E, Bacsadi A, et al. Encephalitis due to West Nile virus in a sheep. Vet Rec 2007;161:568–9.

18. Tyler JW, Turnquist SE, David AT, et al. West Nile virus encephalomyelitis in a sheep. J Vet Intern Med 2003;17:242–4.

19. Tyler JW, Middleton JR. Transmissible spongiform encephalopathies in ruminants. Vet Clin North Am Food Anim Pract 2004;20:303–26.

20. Prusiner SB. Prions. Proc Natl Acad Sci U S A 1998;95:13363–83.

21. Prusiner SB. The prion diseases. Brain Pathol 1998;8:499–513.

22. Wells GAH, Scott AC, Johnson CT, et al. A novel progressive spongiform encephalopathy in cattle. Vet Rec 1987;121:419–20.

23. Number of reported cases of bovine spongiform encephalopathy (BSE) worldwide. Office International des Epizooties (OIE). 2016. Available at: http://www.oie.int/animal-health-in-the-world/bse-situation-in-the-world-and-annual-incidence-rate/10-13-number-of-reported-cases-worldwide-excluding-the-united-kingdom-copy-1/. Accessed June 24, 2016.

24. Horn G. Review of the origin of BSE. London: Department for Environment, Food and Rural Affairs (DEFRA); 2001. p. 1–69.

25. Phillips N, Bridgeman J, Ferguson-Smith M. The BSE inquiry: the report, vols. 1–16. London: Her Majesty's Stationary Office (HMSO) Publications Centre; 2000.

26. Wilesmith JW, Wells GA. Bovine spongiform encephalopathy. Curr Top Microbiol Immunol 1991;172:21–38.

27. Hoinville LJ. A review of the epidemiology of scrapie in sheep. Rev Sci Tech 1996; 15:827–52.

28. Curnow RN, Hodge A, Wilesmith JW. Analysis of the bovine spongiform encephalopathy maternal cohort study: the discordant case-control pairs. Appl Stat 1997;46:345–9.

29. Donnelly CA, Ghani AC, Ferguson NM, et al. Analysis of the bovine spongiform encephalopathy maternal cohort study: evidence for direct maternal transmission. Appl Stat 1997;46:321–44.

30. Gore SM, Gilks WR, Wilesmith JW. Bovine spongiform encephalopathy maternal cohort study – exploratory analysis. Appl Stat 1997;46:305–20.

31. Guldimann C, Gspone M, Drogemuller, et al. Atypical H-type Bovine Spongiform Encephalopathy in a Cow Born after the Reinforced Feed Ban on Meat-and-Bone Meal in Europe. J Clin Microbiol 2012;50:4171–4.

32. European Commission. Update of the opinion on TSE infectivity distribution in ruminant tissues. Brussels (Belgium): EC, Scientific Steering Committee, Health and Consumer Protection Directorate General; 2002. p. 1–53.

33. Lasmezas CI. Transmissible spongiform encephalopathies. Rev Sci Tech 2003; 22:23–36.

34. Wilesmith JW, Ryan JB, Hueston WD, et al. Bovine spongiform encephalopathy: epidemiologic features 1985-1990. Vet Rec 1992;130:90–4.

35. BSE: how to spot and report the disease. Department for Environment, Food & Rural Affairs and Animal and Plant Agency; 2015. Available at: https://www.gov.uk/guidance/bse. Accessed June 29, 2016.

36. Saegerman C, Claes L, Dewaele A, et al. Differential diagnosis of neurologically expressed disorders in Western European cattle. Rev Sci Tech 2003;22:83–102.

37. Hunter GD. Scrapie. Prog Med Virol 1974;18:289–306.

38. Detwiler LA, Baylis M. The epidemiology of scrapie. Rev Sci Tech 2003;22: 121–43.

39. Wineland NE, Detwiler LA, Salman MD. Epidemiologic analysis of reported scrapie in sheep in the United States: 1,117 cases (1947-1992). J Am Vet Med Assoc 1998;212:1537–8.

40. Sweeney T, Hanrahan JP. The evidence of associations between prion protein genotype and production, reproduction, and health traits in sheep. Vet Res 2008;39:28.

41. Scrapie sample submission. United States Department of Agriculture, Animal and Plant Health Inspection Service. 2015. Available at: https://www.aphis.usda.gov/aphis/ourfocus/animalhealth/animal-disease-information/sheep-and-goat-health/national-scrapie-eradication-program/ct_app-labs-genotype-test/!ut/p/z1/hVHR colwEPwaH_EuITWhb2AZsbUyoyKSI45CRKZIHKRS_75onc44Vszb5XZv925Bwg JksTxk6bLKdLHMmzqSvY8x6Q9QMDIauC8Ebc8avnm8h74wITwDRj7rE2eKI3_u9dB2Z8FsLIgztCjIqzZznaY94e-uO6Q4oRc-3nk2PuLPIXIg-ia5SezLsBa3slOrBN mqR8wbwO2-j0SixiS_a9InEB4yVUNQ6HLbJDA9TdzFWQIRZ3xIJdQ0EkKUwQ SnhsWeuJFQXBOIaMLiGDyE17OFttD6fyeT5ARPc736TdsuVqZIQZZqrUpVdr_K5ntTVbv9cwc7WNd1N9U6zVU31tsO_kfZ6H0Fi2sk7LZBUByNz4moZ-tNLo5 mnv4Aaq3Mjg!!/dz/d5/L2dBISEvZ0FBIS9nQSEh/?urile=wcm%3Apath%3A%2Faphis_content_library%2Fsa_our_focus%2Fsa_animal_health%2Fsa_animal_disease_information%2Fsa_sheep_goat_health%2Fsa_scrapie%2Fct_app-labs-genotype-test. Accessed June 29, 2016.

42. Williams ES, Young S. Spongiform encephalopathies in Cervidae. Rev Sci Tech 1992;11:551–67.
43. Chronic wasting disease. Centers for Disease Control and Prevention; 2015. Available at: http://www.cdc.gov/prions/cwd/index.html. Accessed June 29, 2016.
44. Chronic wasting disease. United States Geological Survey, National Wildlife Health Center; 2015. Available at: http://www.nwhc.usgs.gov/disease_informa tion/chronic_wasting_disease/. Accessed June 29, 2016.
45. Mackay RJ, Van Metre DC. Diseases of the nervous system. In: Smith BP, editor. Large animal internal medicine. 5th edition. St Louis (MO): Elsevier Mosby; 2015. p. 923, 943, 948–54, 959–61, 964.
46. Nagy DW. Parelaphostrongylus tenuis and other parasitic diseases of the ruminant nervous system. Vet Clin North Am Food Anim Pract 2004;20:393–412.
47. Foreign animal diseases, 7th edition. Committee on foreign animal diseases of the United States animal health association. St Joseph (MO): USAHA; 2008. p. 147–58, 167–74, 287–96, 321–4, 401–4, 405–10.
48. Smith MO, George LW. Brain tumors. In: Smith BP, editor. Large animal internal medicine. 5th edition. St Louis (MO): Elsevier Mosby; 2015. p. 932–3.
49. Fournier D, Keppie N, Simko E. Bovine familial convulsions and ataxia in Saskatchewan and Alberta. Can Vet J 2004;45:845–8.

Cerebellar Disease of Ruminants

Philippa Gibbons, BVetMed(Hons), MS, MRCVS

KEYWORDS

- Cerebellar hypoplasia • Cerebellar abiotrophy • Lysosomal storage disease

KEY POINTS

- The cerebellum functions to regulate and coordinate motor activity.
- Clinical signs of cerebellar disease include hypermetric gait in all limbs, normal to increased muscle tone, wide-based stance, swaying (truncal ataxia), and intention tremor. Vestibular signs may be observed.
- Cerebellar hypoplasia is most commonly caused by viral disease, and animals are affected from birth.
- Cerebellar abiotrophy is most often heritable, and offspring are typically born normal and develop neurologic signs later in life.
- Plant toxicities and congenital lysosomal storage disorders are differentials for cerebellar disease.

INTRODUCTION AND ANATOMY OF THE CEREBELLUM

The cerebellum is composed of several distinct areas. Knowledge of the anatomy is important when attempting to localize a lesion in the cerebellum. There is a central median region (also called the vermis) with lateral hemispheres on either side. The flocculonodular lobe (the vestibular cerebellum) is located on the ventral, central aspect of the cerebellum. Three cerebellar peduncles attach the cerebellum to the brainstem. The peduncles attach in a caudal to rostral position: the spinal cord and medulla, the pons, and the mesencephalon, respectively. The cerebellar medulla is composed of white matter and surrounded by the cerebellar cortex. The cerebellum receives afferent input from the cerebral cortex and brain stem, vestibular centers, and spinocerebellar pathways. Efferent pathways connect to the brain stem and cerebrocortical areas via Purkinje fibers.[1] The primary function of the cerebellum is to regulate and coordinate motor activity.[1,2]

The author has nothing to disclose.
Food Animal Medicine, Large Animal Clinical Sciences, Texas A&M University, College of Veterinary Medicine and Biomedical Sciences, TAMU 4475, College Station, TX 77845, USA
E-mail address: Pgibbons@cvm.tamu.edu

CLINICAL PRESENTATION OF CEREBELLAR DISEASE

Clinical signs of cerebellar disease vary depending on the location of the disease process within the cerebellum, although diffuse disease is common. Clinical signs characteristic of cerebellar disease include bilaterally symmetric ataxia without paresis and with normal to increased muscle tone. Where there are unilateral lesions, ataxia will be seen on the ipsilateral side to the lesion. Classically the animal will display a hypermetric gait in all 4 limbs, whereby voluntary movement is exaggerated. The animal may stand with a wide-based stance and sway from side to side while ambulating (truncal ataxia). If the cerebellar cortex is affected, a head intention tremor is observed. The intention tremor may cease when the animal is recumbent and muscles are relaxed.[3] In severe disease, the animal may be in lateral recumbency and unable to right itself and display opisthotonus (where the rostral lobe is involved). When performing a neurologic examination, postural reactions may be delayed and then exaggerated. Nystagmus may be present, with variable directions observed when the head is moved.[2] Abnormal menace reaction may also be present[1] with the head moving away from the threatening gesture, but no blink reflex is observed. Neurologic signs may be enhanced if the animal is suddenly released from restraint, which may be observed as cerebellar convulsions.[1] If the flocculonodular lobe is affected, vestibular signs may be apparent, including head tilt and leaning and falling to the contralateral side of the lesion.[1]

DISEASES OF THE CEREBELLUM
Differentiating Cerebellar Abiotrophy and Hypoplasia

Cerebellar abiotrophy occurs because of a variety of familial diseases. Typically, the animal will be born neurologically normal, with the clinical signs developing at weeks to months of age. The cerebellum may be small on necropsy in abiotrophy cases; however, typically it is normal in size. A small cerebellum is found grossly with cerebellar hypoplasia. In abiotrophy cases, the Purkinje cells in the cerebellar cortex are degenerate.[4] In hypoplasia cases, animals are affected from birth, most commonly as a result of viral disease contracted during gestation. Ratio of the cerebellum to whole brain weight can confirm hypoplasia.[4]

Viral-Induced Cerebellar Disease

Cerebellar hypoplasia has been reported in cases of experimental[5] and natural exposure of pregnant cattle to bovine viral diarrhea virus (BVDV).[6] Congenital abnormalities of BVDV (both cerebellar hypoplasia and ocular abnormalities) occur following infection of the cow at 125 to 180 days in gestation. Administration of a modified live BVDV vaccine induced teratogenesis during 90 to 118 days' gestation.[7] Clinical signs of cerebellar disease may be variable in affected calves, from mild to severe.[8] Cerebellar hypoplasia has been recognized as part of the congenital defects associated with the sheep *Pestivirus* (border disease virus)[9] and experimental infection of ewes with BVDV virus.[10] Precolostral serum of calves born with congenital cerebellar infection as a result of BVD had BVD antibody[11] and testing calves before consumption of colostrum may be helpful in the diagnosis of congenital BVD infection.

Schmallenberg virus was first recognized in Northern Europe in 2011 when malformed calves, lambs, and kids were born. Gross lesions recognized included porencephaly, hydraencephaly, cerebellar dysplasia, dysplasia of the brainstem and spinal cord, brachygnathia inferior, arthrogryposis, and vertebral column malformations. Some cases also showed encephalomyelitis. Ninety-five percent of lambs and 45% of calves affected in the Netherlands had cerebellar dysplasia of varying degrees.[12] Microscopically, the cerebellar cortex was affected with loss of Purkinje cells and depletion of the granular layer.[12] *Culicoides* spp midges were determined to be the vector involved in the spread of Schmallenberg virus. Brain lesions were observed when fetuses were infected during 60 to 180 days' gestation in cattle.[8] Bluetongue virus, an *Orbivirus*, is also spread by *Culicoides* spp midges. Cerebellar defects with bluetongue are usually observed in conjunction with other deformities[13] and depend on the serotype.[8,14] Some of the *Orthobunyaviruses* have been associated with cerebellar hypoplasia in cattle. The arthropod-borne Aino virus has been implicated in causing arthrogryposis, hydraencephaly, and cerebellar hypoplasia syndrome in Japanese calves whose dams were inoculated with the virus at 132 to 156 days' gestation.[15–17] Cerebellar hypoplasia was not recognized in goats and cattle experimentally infected with Akabane virus[18]; however, polymyositis and nonpurulent encephalomyelitis were found in calf fetuses of animals inoculated with the virus at 2 to 6 months of gestation. The Chuzan virus found in Japan is related to the Aino and Akabane viruses[8] and has been associated with hydraencephaly cerebellar hypoplasia syndrome.[19] Other viruses that have been implicated in cases of cerebellar disease include a divergent astrovirus found in cases of neuronal necrosis, microgliosis, and perivascular cuffing in the gray matter of the cerebellum.[14]

Congenital Cerebellar Hypoplasia

Familial cerebellar hypoplasia has been reported in Hereford,[16,17] Shorthorns,[17,20] and Ayrshire calves.[21] A congenital cause was also presumed for hypoplasia found in Jersey calves, although calves also had precolostral BVD antibodies, which may have confounded the diagnosis.[22] Hypoplasia in a Japanese shorthorn calf was found in conjunction with Arnold-Chiari malformation.[23] Weaver syndrome (bovine progressive degenerative myeloencephalopathy), recognized in Brown Swiss cattle, shows changes histopathologically to the Purkinje layer of the cerebellum as well as abnormalities in skeletal muscle, reproductive tracts, and white matter of the spinal cord at all levels.[24]

Cerebellar Abiotrophy

In cases of neurogenetic cerebellar abiotrophy, there are rarely apparent gross lesions; but loss of Purkinje cells, swollen axons in the granular layer, and accumulation of glial cells are apparent histologically.[25] The disease has been recognized in Angus calves 2 to 24 months old[25,26] and in poll Hereford cross calves between birth and 8 months old.[17,27] Other breeds whereby cerebellar abiotrophy has been reported include Ayrshires, Charolais,[28] shorthorns, and Limousin.[3] In Holsteins in Brazil, calves were reportedly affected from birth, with most calves lost by 6 months old.[29] The neurogenetic condition bovine familial convulsions and ataxia in Angus cattle has been reported in the United Kingdom, United States, and Canada.[30] Calves were reportedly affected from 4 days to 3 months of age. In this syndrome, axonal swelling of the Purkinje cells was observed histologically.[31] A similar presentation of disease was also observed in a Charolais[32] and poll Hereford and crossbred Angus calves.[3] Calves showed signs of cerebellar disorder and tetanic seizures induced by excitation[3] that lasted several hours in duration, with the frequency decreasing with age in some animals. Merino sheep at least 3.5 years or older have been reported showing progressive clinical signs consistent with cerebellar disease and with histopathologic signs consistent with cerebellar abiotropy.[33] Cerebellar abiotrophy has also been reported in Wiltshire sheep; however, in this breed, young lambs were affected.[34] A similar presenting cerebellar disease in sheep has been recognized in England and Canada and termed daft lamb disease. At necropsy, these lambs had cerebellar atrophy. The hereditability of this disease is unknown and has been observed in multiple breeds.[35]

However, other reports of similar clinical presentations failed to show cerebellar pathology.[36]

Hereditary neuraxial edema (also termed congenital myoclonus or Doddler syndrome) has been observed in Hereford cattle.[3] Calves were affected from birth and displayed tonic-clonic contractions with apnea followed by dyspnea when stimulated.[3] Grossly, the brain appeared normal, with vacuolation (edema) of the cerebellum histologically.[37]

Hereditary hypermetria has been recognized in shorthorn cattle in Brazil, where calves were affected from birth. The disease was observed in a herd where an affected bull was used and suggested an autosomal recessive mode of inheritance. Pathologically this disease appeared different from both abiotrophy and hypoplasia.[29]

Transmissible Spongiform Encephalopathies

Degeneration and vacuolation of Purkinje cells in the cerebellum of sheep has been reported in cases of natural transmission of scrapie.[38] The consistency and severity of lesions in the cerebellum was reported to differ between breeds of sheep.[39]

Plant Toxicities

Solanum species of plants have been found to cause cerebellar disease in both cattle and goats. Species include *Solanum viarum*[40] in Florida, *Solanum kwebense* in South Africa,[41] *Solanum bonariense* in Uruguay,[42] and *Solanum subinerme* in Brazil.[43] In affected goats, histopathologic lesions were observed throughout the cerebellum consistent with a storage disease; however, the mechanism of the toxicity is unknown. No other brain lesions have been observed with *Solanum* toxicity, and clinically affected animals failed to respond once removed from the environment.[40] Experimental ingestion of this plant produced clinical signs after 128 days at a threshold dose of 1.024 kg/kg body mass.[42] Lesions observed histologically in *Solanum* toxicities are of wallerian-type degeneration of the cerebellum alone,[42] with loss of Purkinje cells.[41,44] *Solanum* species of plants are found across the United States. The source of the toxicity (fruit, leaf, or stems) is unknown.

Astragalus, *Oxytropis*, and *Swainsona* species of plants can also cause cerebellar disease as a result of inhibition of lysosomal enzymes (alpha-D-mannosidase and Golgi mannosidase II), resulting in accumulation of their substrates. These plants are collectively known as locoweeds. These plants are documented worldwide. In the United States, distribution of *Oxytropis* and *Astragalus* species is primarily in the West and Southwest.[45] *Ipomoea* spp have been reported to be found in Brazil[46] and Mozambique[47] and cause neurologic disease. Younger animals are commonly more affected, and neurologic lesions are not limited to the cerebellum.[45] Recovery of the affected animals can occur once removed from the plant source, although neurologic deficits may remain.

LYSOSOMAL STORAGE DISEASES

Congenital lysosomal storage diseases in cattle that have been reported to present with cerebellar signs include alpha-mannosidosis of Angus, Murray Grey, square meter (Angus-derived composite breed), and Galloway breeds; beta-mannosidosis in Salers; and maple syrup urine disease in poll Herefords and poll shorthorns.[25]

Maple syrup urine disease is an autosomal recessive disorder. A branched-chain ketoacid dehydrogenase deficiency causes an accumulation of branched-chain keto acids and their precursor amino acids.[48] The location of the mutation for this disease has been detected.[49] Affected calves are initially normal at birth with rapid deterioration and death. The urine has a strong smell described as curry or maple syrup. Pathology described includes changes in the white matter of the cerebrum, cerebellum, midbrain, and hindbrain.[25]

Alpha-mannosidosis is also inherited as an autosomal recessive trait.[50] Calves have a deficiency of alpha-mannosidase enzyme, which results in nonlipid vacuolation of cells in the cerebrum, cerebellum, and spinal nerves.[31] Calves are typically born neurologically normal, with clinical signs consistent with cerebellar disease developing over months. However, the disease reported in Galloway calves was detected in stillborn or aborted calves.[51] Affected calves are usually small and may have secondary disease. The disease has been recognized in Angus cattle in the United Kingdom, United States, and Australia.[52]

Beta-mannosidosis has been reported in Salers calves and affects them from birth and is suspected to be an autosomal recessive trait.[53] Vacuolation of the Purkinje cells and decreased myelination of the cerebellum is observed, along with changes in other areas of the brain, renal, thyroid, and lymphoid tissue.[53] Beta-mannosidosis has also been reported in Nubian goats.[54,55]

Other lysosomal storage diseases of cattle affecting the nervous system include GM1 gangliosidosis of Friesian cattle, characterized by forebrain disease and stunted growth[56] occurring within the first month of life.[56] Ocular lesions may also be seen,[57] and the disease has also been reported in sheep.[58] Pompe disease (glycogen storage disease II) has been recognized in shorthorn and Brahman cattle, resulting in incoordination, stunted growth, and muscle weakness causing recumbency.[25] Glycogen storage disease 5 in Charolais affects muscles, and citrullinemia in Holstein-Friesians causes cerebral disease secondary to hyperammonemia.[25]

OTHER CAUSES OF TREMORS IN RUMINANTS

Other conditions causing tremors, which may be confused with cerebellar disease, include grass staggers and hypomagnesemia. Perennial ryegrass (*Lolium* spp) is affected with *Acremonium* spp of fungus. The fungal toxin acts at the γ-aminobutyric acid receptors[3] and results in neurologic lesions consistent with cerebellar localization. Histologically, loss of Purkinje cells has been seen in the cerebellum.[45,59] The disease has been observed in North and South America, Australia, and Europe. Bermuda grass (*Cynodon dactylon*), Dallis grass and Canary grass (*Phalaris* spp) can also produce staggerlike signs indistinguishable from ryegrass staggers. *Penicillium* fungus found on moldy corn stalks can produce tremorogenic mycotoxins, and *Aspergillus clavatus* found on feed also produce similar signs.[3]

REFERENCES

1. Mayhew J. Incoordination of the head and limbs: cerebellar diseases. Large animal neurology. 2nd edition. Chichester (United Kingdom): Wiley-Blackwell; 2008. p. 143–5.
2. De Lahunta A. Cerebellum. In: DeLahunta A, editor. Veterinary neuroanatomy and clinical neurology. Philadelphia: Saunders; 1977. p. 238–56.
3. MacKay RJ, Van Meter DC. Large animal internal medicine. 5th edition. St Louis (MO): Elsevier Mosby; 2015.
4. Scarratt WK. Cerebellar disease and disease characterized by dysmetria or tremors. Vet Clin North Am Food Anim Pract 2004;20:275–86.
5. Brown TT, DeLahunta A, Bistner SI, et al. Pathogenetic studies of infection of the bovine fetus with bovine viral diarrhea virus. Cerebellar atrophy. Vet Pathol 1974; 11:486–505.

6. Kahrs RF, Scott FW, De Lahunta A. Epidemiological observations on bovine viral diarrhea-mucosal disease virus-induced congenital cerebellar hypoplasia and ocular defects in calves. Teratology 1970;3:181–4.
7. Trautwein G, Hewicker M, Liess B, et al. Studies on transplacental transmissibility of a bovine virus diarrhoea (BVD) vaccine virus in cattle. Occurrence of central nervous system malformations in calves born from vaccinated cows. Zentralbl Veterinarmed B 1986;33:260–8.
8. Agerholm JS, Hewicker-Trautwein M, Peperkamp K, et al. Virus-induced congenital malformations in cattle. Acta Vet Scand 2015;57:54.
9. Barlow RM. Morphogenesis of hydranencephaly and other intracranial malformations in progeny of pregnant ewes infected with pestiviruses. J Comp Pathol 1980;90:87–98.
10. Gruber AD, Hewicker-Trautwein M, Liess B, et al. Brain malformations in ovine fetuses associated with the cytopathogenic biotype of bovine viral-diarrhoea virus. Zentralbl Veterinarmed B 1995;42:443–7.
11. Kahrs RF, Scott FW, De Lahunta A. Congenital cerebella hypoplasia and ocular defects in calves following bovine viral diarrhea-mucosal disease infection in pregnant cattle. J Am Vet Med Assoc 1970;156:1443–50.
12. Peperkamp NH, Luttikholt SJ, Dijkman R, et al. Ovine and bovine congenital abnormalities associated with intrauterine infection with Schmallenberg virus. Vet Pathol 2015;52:1057–66.
13. Wouda W, Peperkamp NH, Roumen MP, et al. Epizootic congenital hydranencephaly and abortion in cattle due to bluetongue virus serotype 8 in the Netherlands. Tijdschr Diergeneeskd 2009;134:422–7.
14. Li L, Diab S, McGraw S, et al. Divergent astrovirus associated with neurologic disease in cattle. Emerg Infect Dis 2013;19:1385–92.
15. Tsuda T, Yoshida K, Ohashi S, et al. Arthrogryposis, hydranencephaly and cerebellar hypoplasia syndrome in neonatal calves resulting from intrauterine infection with Aino virus. Vet Res 2004;35:531–8.
16. Innes JRM, Russell DS, Wilsdon AJ. Familial cerebellar hypoplasia and degeneration in Hereford calves. J Pathol 1940;50:455–61.
17. Hulland TJ. Cerebellar ataxia in calves. Can J Comp Med Vet Sci 1957;21:72–6.
18. Konno S, Nakagawa M. Akabane disease in cattle: congenital abnormalities caused by viral infection. Experimental disease. Vet Pathol 1982;19:267–79.
19. Miura Y, Kubo M, Goto Y, et al. Hydranencephaly-cerebellar hypoplasia in a newborn calf after infection of its dam with Chuzan virus. Nihon Juigaku Zasshi 1990;52:689–94.
20. Swan RA, Taylor EG. Cerebellar hypoplasia in beef shorthorn calves. Aust Vet J 1982;59:95–6.
21. Howell JM, Ritchie HE. Cerebellar malformations in two Ayrshire calves. Pathol Vet 1966;3:159–68.
22. Allen JG. Congenital cerebellar hypoplasia in Jersey calves. Aust Vet J 1977;53:173–5.
23. Madarame H, Azuma K, Nozuki H, et al. Cerebellar hypoplasia associated with Arnold-Chiari malformation in a Japanese shorthorn calf. J Comp Pathol 1991;104:1–5.
24. Stuart LD, Leipold HW. Lesions in bovine progressive degenerative myeloencephalopathy ("weaver") of brown Swiss cattle. Vet Pathol 1985;22:13–23.
25. Windsor P, Kessell A, Finnie J. Neurological diseases of ruminant livestock in Australia. V: congenital neurogenetic disorders of cattle. Aust Vet J 2011;89:394–401.

26. Mitchell PJ, Reilly W, Harper PA, et al. Cerebellar abiotrophy in Angus cattle. Aust Vet J 1993;70:67–8.

27. Whittington RJ, Morton AG, Kennedy DJ. Cerebellar abiotrophy in crossbred cattle. Aust Vet J 1989;66:12–5.

28. de Lahunta A. Abiotrophy in domestic animals: a review. Can J Vet Res 1990;54:65–76.

29. Schild AL, Riet-Correa F, Portiansky EL, et al. Congenital cerebellar cortical degeneration in Holstein cattle in Southern Brazil. Vet Res Commun 2001;25:189–95.

30. Fournier D, Keppie N, Simko E. Bovine familial convulsions and ataxia in Saskatchewan and Alberta. Can Vet J 2004;45:845–8.

31. Barlow RM. Morphogenesis of cerebellar lesions in bovine familial convulsions and ataxia. Vet Pathol 1981;18:151–62.

32. Cho DY, Leipold HW. Cerebellar cortical atrophy in a Charolais calf. Vet Pathol 1978;15:264–6.

33. Harper PA, Duncan DW, Plant JW, et al. Cerebellar abiotrophy and segmental axonopathy: two syndromes of progressive ataxia of Merino sheep. Aust Vet J 1986;63:18–21.

34. Johnstone AC, Johnson CB, Malcolm KE, et al. Cerebellar cortical abiotrophy in Wiltshire sheep. N Z Vet J 2005;53:242–5.

35. Innes JR, MacNaughton. Inherited cortical cerebellar atrophy in Corriedale lambs in Canada identical with "daft lamb" disease in Britain. Cornell Vet 1950;40:127–35.

36. Terlecki S, Richardson C, Bradley R, et al. A congenital disease of lambs clinically similar to 'inherited cerebellar cortical atrophy' (daft lamb disease). Br Vet J 1978;134:299–307.

37. Cordy DR, Richards WP, Stormont C. Hereditary neuraxial edema in Hereford calves. Pathol Vet 1969;6:487–501.

38. Zlotnik I. Cerebellar and midbrain lesions in scrapie. Nature 1960;185:785.

39. Wood JL, McGill IS, Done SH, et al. Neuropathology of scrapie: a study of the distribution patterns of brain lesions in 222 cases of natural scrapie in sheep, 1982-1991. Vet Rec 1997;140:167–74.

40. Porter MB, MacKay RJ, Uhl E, et al. Neurologic disease putatively associated with ingestion of Solanum viarum in goats. J Am Vet Med Assoc 2003;223:501–4, 456.

41. van der Lugt JJ, Bastianello SS, van Ederen AM, et al. Cerebellar cortical degeneration in cattle caused by Solanum kwebense. Vet J 2010;185:225–7.

42. Verdes JM, Morana A, Gutierrez F, et al. Cerebellar degeneration in cattle grazing Solanum bonariense ("Naranjillo") in Western Uruguay. J Vet Diagn Invest 2006;18:299–303.

43. Lima EF, Riet-Correa F, de Medeiros RM. Spontaneous poisoning by Solanum subinerme Jack as a cause of cerebellar cortical degeneration in cattle. Toxicon 2014;82:93–6.

44. Verdes JM, Marquez M, Calliari A, et al. A novel pathogenic mechanism for cerebellar lesions produced by Solanum bonariense in cattle. J Vet Diagn Invest 2015;27:278–86.

45. Plumlee KH. Clinical veterinary toxicology. St. Louis (MO): Mosby; 2004.

46. Mendonca FS, Albuquerque RF, Evencio-Neto J, et al. Alpha-mannosidosis in goats caused by the swainsonine-containing plant Ipomoea verbascoidea. J Vet Diagn Invest 2012;24:90–5.

47. de Balogh KK, Dimande AP, van der Lugt JJ, et al. A lysosomal storage disease induced by Ipomoea carnea in goats in Mozambique. J Vet Diagn Invest 1999;11: 266–73.

48. Healy PJ, Dennis JA, Harper PA, et al. Maple syrup urine disease in poll shorthorn calves. Aust Vet J 1992;69:143–4.

49. Dennis JA, Healy PJ. Definition of the mutation responsible for maple syrup urine disease in poll shorthorns and genotyping poll shorthorns and poll Herefords for maple syrup urine disease alleles. Res Vet Sci 1999;67:1–6.

50. Jolly RD, Thompson KG. The pathology of bovine mannosidosis. Vet Pathol 1978; 15:141–52.

51. Embury DH, Jerrett IV. Mannosidosis in Galloway calves. Vet Pathol 1985;22: 548–51.

52. Leipold HW, Smith JE, Jolly RD, et al. Mannosidosis of Angus calves. J Am Vet Med Assoc 1979;175:457–9.

53. Bryan L, Schmutz S, Hodges SD, et al. Bovine beta-mannosidosis: pathologic and genetic findings in Salers calves. Vet Pathol 1993;30:130–9.

54. Lovell KL, Kranich RJ, Cavanagh KT. Biochemical and histochemical analysis of lysosomal enzyme activities in caprine beta-mannosidosis. Mol Chem Neuropathol 1994;21:61–74.

55. Leipprandt JR, Kraemer SA, Haithcock BE, et al. Caprine beta-mannosidase: sequencing and characterization of the cDNA and identification of the molecular defect of caprine beta-mannosidosis. Genomics 1996;37:51–6.

56. Donnelly WJ, Sheahan BJ, Kelly M. Beta-galactosidase deficiency in GM1 gangliosidosis of Friesian calves. Res Vet Sci 1973;15:139–41.

57. Sheahan BJ, Donnelly WJ, Grimes TD. Ocular pathology of bovine GM1 gangliosidosis. Acta Neuropathol 1978;41:91–5.

58. Skelly BJ, Jeffrey M, Franklin RJ, et al. A new form of ovine GM1-gangliosidosis. Acta Neuropathol 1995;89:374–9.

59. Oz HH, Nicholson SS, Al-Bagdadi FK, et al. Cerebellar disease in an adult cow. Can Vet J 1986;27:13–6.

Brainstem and Cranial Nerve Disorders of Ruminants

Mélanie J. Boileau, DVM, MS*, John Gilliam, DVM, MS*

KEYWORDS

- Brainstem • Cranial nerves • Ruminant • Listeriosis • Otitis media/interna
- Pituitary abscess

KEY POINTS

- Listeriosis, otitis/media interna, and pituitary abscess syndrome are the most common causes of asymmetrical brainstem abnormalities in ruminants.
- Differentiation of these diseases can usually be made based on typical clinical and neurologic signs, and historical findings.
- Laboratory diagnostics such as blood work and cerebrospinal fluid analysis may be supportive, but do not provide a definitive diagnosis because of variation and overlap in the typical findings.
- Presumptive diagnosis is usually based on clinical and neurologic signs, and confirmed at necropsy.
- Treatment involves a prolonged course of antibiotic therapy but is unrewarding in cases of pituitary abscess syndrome.

LISTERIOSIS

Listeriosis is the designated term for infections associated with *Listeria monocytogenes.* The organism is shed in the feces and thus is ubiquitous in the environment. The disease has a worldwide distribution, occurs most often in temperate climates and affects a wide range of mammals including ruminants, monogastric animals and humans. In ruminants, *L monocytogenes* causes neurologic disease (encephalitic listeriosis), keratoconjunctivitis, septicemia, mastitis, abortion, and diarrhea. Encephalitic listeriosis is the most common form. Encephalitic listeriosis is mostly sporadic and often associated with winter housing and ingestion of poorly preserved silage. Neurologic listeriosis may manifest as a multifocal brainstem disorder, diffuse

The authors have nothing to disclose.
Veterinary Clinical Sciences, College of Veterinary Medicine, Oklahoma State University, 2065 West Farm Road, Stillwater, OK 74078-2041, USA
* Corresponding author.
E-mail addresses: melanie.boileau@okstate.edu; john.gilliam@okstate.edu

vetfood.theclinics.com

meningoencephalitis, or myelitis. The presumptive diagnosis can be made based on neurologic signs and cerebrospinal fluid (CSF) analysis. Definitive diagnosis is made at necropsy. Antibiotic treatment can be effective if initiated early, but the case fatality rate is high, especially in small ruminants. Listeriosis is also a zoonosis and may occur either after direct contact with affected animals or more frequently as foodborne disease.

Etiology

L monocytogenes is a small, non–spore-forming, facultative anaerobic, gram-positive rod. L monocytogenes is found worldwide and is widely distributed in the environment. The reservoirs of infection are the soil and the intestinal tracts of humans, as well as domesticated and wild mammals, birds, fish, and crustaceans.[1,2] Carrier animals are usually asymptomatic.[3] Infected animals can shed L monocytogenes in the feces, milk, and uterine discharges. Soil or fecal contamination results in its presence on plants and in silage. L monocytogenes is resistant to adverse environmental conditions. It may persist for months to years in soil, bedding, silages, fecal material, water, and contaminated feed.[1]

The bacterium can tolerate a wide range of pH and temperatures. Optimum growth occurs at 30°C to 37°C but the organism can multiply at 4°C to 45°C. One of the unique characteristic of L monocytogenes is its ability to replicate at refrigeration temperature (4° to 6°C).[4,5] L monocytogenes can multiply within a wide range of pH (5.6–9.6) but is inhibited by a pH of less than 5.6.[2]

L monocytogenes is a facultative intracellular bacterium that is capable of multiplying in macrophages and monocytes, which contributes to its pathogenicity and to a poor response to antibiotic therapy. Bacterial virulence factors produced by L monocytogenes that are necessary for adhesion, intracellular multiplication, and overall pathogenicity include hemolysin, listeriolysin O, phospholipases, the protein ActA, and internalins.[6,7] There are many serotypes of L monocytogenes, but serotypes 1/2a and 4b are the major contributors to encephalitic listeriosis of ruminants,[8] with serotype 1/2b isolated in a small proportion of cases.[2,9,10]

Epidemiology

Listeriosis has a worldwide distribution, but occurs most often in temperate climates. In ruminants, various forms of listeriosis are described. They include a neurologic form (multifocal brainstem disorder, diffuse meningoencephalitis or myelitis), an ocular form (keratoconjunctivitis and uveitis with or without hypopyon, commonly referred to as "silage eye"),[3,11] a septicemic form (neonatal death), a reproductive form (sporadic late-term abortion), a mammary form (mastitis), and a gastroenteritis form (diarrhea).[12]

Encephalitic listeriosis is the most common clinical manifestation of listeriosis in ruminants.[10,13] Encephalitic listeriosis occurs worldwide and is reported more frequently in sheep and cattle than in goats.[14,15] There is no sex predilection. Any breed of ruminant can be affected; however, 2 individual studies have suggested an increased risk in Rambouillet sheep[16] and Angora goats.[17]

Animals of all ages are susceptible to encephalitic listeriosis, with ruminant cases reported as early as the first month of life[9,18,19] to as late as 9[20,21] or 10 years of age.[22] Younger animals are affected at times corresponding with tooth loss or eruption of the permanent teeth.[18,19] Encephalitic listeriosis is rare in calves less than 6 months of age.[15] Occurrences in nursing and weaned lambs,[9,18,19] feedlot cattle,[23] browsing goats,[8,17] lactating dairy cows,[23] and camelids[24,25] illustrate the diversity of susceptibility.[15] In some reports, a single age group or single location on a farm is affected whereas in others, infection spans a wide age range or several locations. These differences are probably a result of the source, location, extent, and duration of *L monocytogenes* exposure.[15]

The incidence and prevalence of encephalitic listeriosis are not well-documented. Encephalitic listeriosis can affect a single animal within a herd,[21,26,27] but most reports involve multiple cases over a short period of time. Within a herd, the encephalitic form of listeriosis is typically sporadic, with a prevalence of less than 5%.[19,23,28,29] Outbreaks of encephalitic listeriosis are usually observed in sheep, in which the incidence of disease may range between 8% and 34%.[30–33] In contrast, the incidence of listeriosis outbreaks in cattle is lower, affecting 10% or less of the animals in the herd on average.[34] One study reported that the incidence of clinically apparent encephalitic listeriosis in dairy cows and replacement heifers in England was 11 and 67 per 1000 cows per year, respectively, in affected herds compared with 0.25 and 0.31 per 1000 cows per year, respectively, in all herds.[34] Overall, the disease in sheep and goats tends to be more acute and results in higher morbidity and mortality than in cattle.[8,35]

Clinical cases of encephalitic listeriosis can occur at any time of the year, but are more frequent in late winter[9,26,29,31,34,36,37] or early spring.[18] Moreover, in cattle, sheep, and goats, the prevalence of *L monocytogenes* in fecal samples peaks during winter.[8,14,37,38] Reasons to explain this seasonal variation include housing of animals,[39] which increases stocking density and fecal contamination of the environment, feeding poor quality feed that has been stored, particularly silage, and stress and/or immune deficiency associated with concurrent diseases[30] and adverse weather conditions.[15,31] Outbreaks of listeriosis have been reported after periods of very heavy rain.[30,40]

Risk Factors

In ruminants, the most widely accepted risk factor for encephalitic listeriosis is consumption of poorly preserved and bacteriologically contaminated silage.[15] Circumstantial evidence includes development of encephalitic listeriosis shortly after the onset of silage feeding,[29,32] resolution of listeriosis outbreaks after cessation of silage feeding,[29,32] and the well-documented higher incidence of encephalitic listeriosis during winter or early spring, when animals are housed and fed silage.[14]

All types of silage are equally prone to *Listeria* contamination.[41] The quality of the silage is also important. The type of silage (ie, grass silage,[28] corn silage,[23] sorghum silage,[23] barley silage,[42] or clover baylage[28]) does not seem to be as important as the preservation condition of the silage. Although *L monocytogenes* can be cultured from well-preserved high-quality silage (pH 4–4.5) in low numbers,[43] the culture rate is much higher in inadequately preserved silage that has a pH greater than 5.5 and/or in which anaerobic conditions are not achieved.[43–46] Silages with poor nutritional value have also been associated with encephalitic listeriosis.[14] Best practices for the production of well-preserved silage have been reviewed elsewhere.[15,47,48]

Encephalitic listeriosis may occur with all types of silage storage. Common sources include spoiled silage at the ends of trench silos,[16] decaying forage at the bottom of the feed bunks,[37] or rotting hay at the periphery of the hay stacks.[19,45,49] Big bales of silage (or hay) present also a greater risk for listeria infection, because of lower density and a greater risk for mechanical damage to the plastic covering.[50] In addition, the risk for contamination of silage is higher when it contains soil.[50]

Uncommonly, inadequate fermentation and proliferation of *L monocytogenes* also occurs in upright conventional silos.[23,46] Therefore, the quality and storage conditions of silage should be examined when encephalitic listeriosis occurs. However, even though improperly preserved silage usually looks grossly abnormal (moldy, off-color), it may also appear normal[23] and this poses a challenge in identification of the source of the contamination.[41] In some instances, only part of the silage may be contaminated. Moreover, the delay between contamination and development of clinical signs is usually long (2–6 weeks),[2] such that all the contaminated silage may have been consumed or discarded by the time the diagnosis of encephalitic listeriosis is made.

Not all animals with encephalitic listeriosis have a history of silage consumption. Encephalitic listeriosis has been observed in animals consuming pasture,[30,40,51] hay,[51] and soybean products.[13] Therefore, although ingestion of poorly preserved silage predisposes to encephalitic listeriosis, the condition can be observed in ruminants on many diets. Another potential risk factor for listeriosis is the use of poultry litter for bedding.[52] L monocytogenes also has been isolated from other bedding materials,[19,38,53] soil,[37] water troughs,[38] feed bunks,[38] rotting vegetation,[1] compost piles,[13] and feed-handling equipment.[29] Fecal contamination is the most likely source of environmental L monocytogenes isolates.[37,53]

Last, animals fed hard or coarse feed seem to be at increased risk of developing encephalitic listeriosis. Reportedly, 1 investigator showed that mice fed hard food were more prone to develop experimental encephalitic listeriosis compared with those fed soft food.[54,55] In another study, feeding of rough browse was identified as a risk factor for encephalitic listeriosis in goats.[17]

Pathogenesis

The pathogenesis of encephalitic listeriosis in ruminants is not completely elucidated. It is unclear whether infection of the brain by L monocytogenes occurs hematogenously or by ascending infection from the cranial nerve rootlets.[56] Earlier investigators considered axonal migration as an unlikely mode of pathogenesis because of a lack of nutritional dependency of L monocytogenes for nervous tissue and the ability to produce multifocal brain microabscesses after intravenous or subcutaneous inoculation of the bacteria into susceptible hosts.[57–59] Conversely, other investigators have suggested and demonstrated that ascending infection of L monocytogenes from the cranial nerve rootlets represents the most plausible pathogenesis. Briefly, the pathogen enters the terminal roots of the trigeminal nerve through small wounds in the oropharyngeal cavity, and then migrates intraaxonally to the trigeminal nucleus in the pons of the brainstem.[54,55,60–62]

Support for this mechanism comes from multiple experimental clinical trials. In 1 study, clinical encephalitis developed in 6 of 21 sheep (29%), 20 to 41 days after experimental inoculation with L monocytogenes in the pulp cavity.[18] Two-thirds of the sheep had histologic evidence of listeriosis on the right side of the medulla. Neuritis and perineuritis were found only in the nerves ascending from the inoculation site, with nerve lesions seeming to be more mature than brain lesions. In another study,[55] 36% of goat kids (4 of 11) injected with L monocytogenes in the buccal submucosa developed encephalitis 17 to 28 days after injection; the cellular reaction could be traced along the trigeminal nerve from the lip to the medulla. Similar observations were made when L monocytogenes was inoculated over puncture wounds on the skin and mucous membrane of the lips of mice[55,60] or when injected into the facial muscle or proximal end of cut facial nerves of mice.[63] L monocytogenes has also been observed within neurons and axons of sheep with naturally occurring encephalitic listeriosis.[57]

Recently, Henke and colleagues[62] and Otter and Blakemore[61] demonstrated that L monocytogenes does spread intraaxonally within the brain along interneuronal connections. The efficient spread of L monocytogenes infection in the brainstem can be explained by its ability to survive phagocytosis and the use of its actin tail polymerization machinery to spread from cell to cell.[62] This allows the pathogen to multiply and diffuse within the brain, protected from the host defenses by avoiding contact with the extracellular compartment.[6,61–63] Reportedly, *L monocytogenes* does not seem to have a specific affinity for the trigeminal nerve because lumbar or thoracic myelitis has developed after adjacent subcutaneous[55] or intramuscular[63] inoculation of *L monocytogenes* in mice. Host and bacterial factors involved in the pathogenesis of listeriosis have been reviewed elsewhere.[15,64,65] Experimental models suggest that clinical signs of encephalitic listeriosis develop 3 to 6 weeks after bacterial inoculation into the oral cavity.[2,18,55]

Clinical Signs

In ruminants, the most common clinical signs associated with *L monocytogenes* infections include encephalitis ("circling disease" or "silage disease"), followed by septicemia in neonates, and sporadic late-term abortions. Other less common manifestations are keratoconjunctivitis with uveitis ("silage eye"), mastitis, and gastroenteritis. Ocular disease associated with *L monocytogenes* may occur in ruminants with no signs of neurologic disease.[11,34,66]

The neurologic signs encountered with encephalitic listeriosis reflect dysfunction of the caudal brainstem, cerebellar peduncles, or less commonly, the spinal cord.[30] Fever may be present early in the clinical course of the disease[22,27,31,35,46] and partial to complete anorexia and depression are also common.[22,67] In some cases, excitement rather than depression has been reported.[32] Heart rate and respiratory rate are variable. Animals may be dehydrated secondary to their inability to swallow. They become unable to drink, and the salivary loss exacerbates the degree of dehydration[41] and may contribute to metabolic acidosis. Rumen contraction rate is usually decreased,[26,35] but rumen hypermotility and projectile vomiting have been reported in cattle with vagal nerve involvement.[21] Bruxism and signs of abdominal pain may be observed as a result of dry rumen contents.[21,34,35]

Central nervous system signs are usually asymmetrical and include conscious proprioceptive deficits, propulsive walking with eventual head pressing when making contact with a solid object,[67] and cranial nerve deficits. Cranial nerve deficits are typically unilateral, but may be bilateral in advanced cases.[22,35] Depression is the result of lesions of the reticular activating system, which can be worsened by severe concurrent metabolic acidosis. Conscious proprioceptive deficits are caused by interference with the descending motor pathways and the ascending proprioceptive fibers in the brainstem[26] and may precede or accompany cranial nerve dysfunction. Propulsive walking or compulsive circling with head pressing are caused by lesions of the basal ganglia.[56]

Cranial nerves V through XII are usually dysfunctional in listeric animals. Patients with loss of the trigeminal nerve (cranial nerve V) function show dropped jaw, poor jaw tone,[26] inability to eat, and facial analgesia or anesthesia.[26,30,35,51,57,58] Facial anesthesia is best detected by stimulation of the nasal septum with a pen or piece of straw.[56] Animals with lesions of the abducens nerve (cranial nerve VI) exhibit a medial strabismus on the ipsilateral side of the lesion. Animals with lesions of the facial nerve (cranial nerve VII) have ipsilateral drooped ear, ptosis, and decreased lip tone.[35,57,58] Decreased motor function of the cranial nerve VII results in loss of menace response, palpebral reflex, and levator nasolabialis muscle function also ipsilaterally. Small ruminants and camelids with cranial nerve VII loss have a deviated nasal philtrum to the opposite side of the lesion. The paralysis of the orbicularis oculi muscle often results in secondary exposure keratitis.[20,35] The loss of levator nasolabialis function is best detected by observation of drooling of saliva from the ipsilateral side of the mouth and by palpation of the lips and nostrils.[56]

Animals with lesions of the vestibulocochlear nerve (cranial nerve VIII) display a nystagmus that changes as the position of the head is altered. The orientation of the nystagmus is variable (mainly horizontal or vertical) and is usually inconsistent.[20,35] Other signs include a head tilt toward the side of the lesion (**Fig. 1**) and a tendency to circle, lean, roll, or fall toward the side of the lesion.[9,22,27,32,35,57,58] In rare instances, paradoxic vestibular syndrome may occur when the cerebellar peduncles are involved, in which case head tilt, circling, and leaning are toward the side contralateral to the lesion.[68] If the spinal reflexes can be tested, affected ruminants with unilateral vestibular lesions show an extensor thrust (hypertonia and hyperreflexia) in the limbs opposite to the side of the lesion, which is most readily apparent in the forelimbs.[15]

Animals with acute loss of glossopharyngeal (cranial nerve IX), vagal (cranial nerve X), and hypoglossal (cranial nerve XII) nerve develop dysphagia, hypersalivation, and, uncommonly, stertorous breathing (cranial nerve X). Affected animals may accumulate feedstuff or rumen cuds into their mouth (see **Fig. 1**) over time, whereas others show reflux of feed through the nose. Severe cases are at increased risk for aspiration pneumonia.[21,27,35] Animals with dysfunctional cranial nerve XII have paresis or paralysis of the tongue[23] (see **Fig. 1**), which contributes to dysphagia. With unilateral lesions, the tongue protrudes from the side of the mouth ipsilateral to the lesion.

Listeric myelitis is not a characteristic sign of encephalitic listeriosis, but has been described in sheep and cattle. The pathologic lesions and clinical signs are restricted

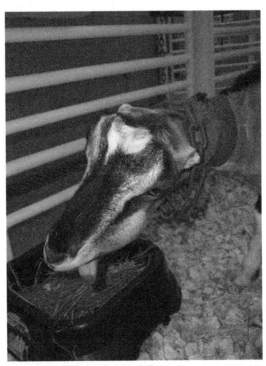

Fig. 1. Three-year-old Lamancha doe with listeriosis. The left-sided head tilt and slight ptosis indicates involvement of the left facial and vestibulocochlear nerve (cranial nerves VII and VIII, respectively). Feed packing in the left cheek and protrusion of the tongue outside the mouth indicates involvement of the left glossopharyngeal and hypoglossal nerve (cranial nerves IX and XII, respectively).

to the spinal cord. Animals affected by listerial myelitis have no apparent brainstem dysfunction but demonstrate paresis or paralysis of 1 or several limbs.[33,40,69]

In the final stages of the disease, severely affected animals become recumbent, unable to rise, and lie on the same side as the lesion.[9,35,67] Some may display torticollis,[32,51] opisthotonos,[23,32,35] or convulsions with propulsive limb movements.[32,35,36] In such cases, prognosis is fatal and affected animals die despite treatment.[22,35] Occasionally, recumbency or death is the first sign observed.[51]

Encephalitic listeriosis progresses more quickly in small ruminants than in cattle. The increased severity of clinical signs coupled with the higher isolation rate of *L monocytogenes* in the brain of small ruminants are hypothesized to be owing to decreased macrophage expression of inducible nitric oxide synthase, compared with that of cattle.[15,70] In sheep and goats, the course of the disease is usually short, with death as soon as 2 to 4 days after appearance of the first clinical signs.[50,71] In cattle, death usually occurs about 2 weeks after the appearance of the first clinical signs.[71] Overall, the case fatality rate is nearly 100% in animals left untreated.

In summary, the neurologic form of listeriosis in ruminants has been called "circling disease" because of the classic involvement of the cranial nerve VII and cranial nerve VIII nuclei that causes facial paresis and propulsive circling toward the affected side.[15] However, because cranial nerve signs can occur in any combination and be unilateral or bilateral, encephalitic listeriosis has a highly variable clinical presentation.

Differentials

In ruminants, the main differential diagnoses for multifocal, particularly unilateral, brainstem disease with inconsistent fever are listeriosis, otitis media (OM)/interna, brainstem abscess or tumors, pituitary abscess syndrome, aberrant parasite migration, and head trauma.[20,68,72] Animals with OM/interna (OMI) are alert, have involvement only of facial and/or vestibulocochlear nerves, and most have otorrhea (references provided elsewhere in this article).[15] Brainstem abscesses and tumors are rare. Trauma often is evident on physical examination or in the history. Aberrant parasite migration usually involves the spinal cord and can be distinguished by eosinophilia in CSF analysis.[15] Animals with pituitary abscess syndrome often are depressed, have a base-wide stance with head and neck extended, bradycardia, or exophthalmia in addition to multiple asymmetrical cranial nerve deficits (references provided elsewhere in this article).[15]

Other neurologic diseases that have been confused with listeriosis are thrombotic meningoencephalitis (*Histophilus somni*), bacterial meningitis (young animals), viral encephalitis (caprine arthritis encephalitis virus, bovine herpesvirus 5, and rabies) and, less commonly, bovine spongiform encephalopathy (in affected countries),[73] polioencephalomalacia (thiamine deficiency), and lead toxicity.

Diagnosis

History (consumption of silage) and classical neurologic signs (multifocal or unilateral brainstem disease) are usually sufficient for a presumptive diagnosis of encephalitic listeriosis.[41] Although complete blood count and serum biochemistry profile are not crucial in the diagnosis of the disease, they are useful indicators of dehydration and the acid–base status of the animal.[20,22,35] A complete blood count can be normal or reflect a stress response or an inflammatory condition. Compared with monogastric species, monocytosis is not observed on complete blood count of ruminants with encephalitic listeriosis.[15] Dehydration and prerenal azotemia may be evaluated by measurement of the hematocrit, total protein concentration, serum creatinine, and blood urea nitrogen values. Many cattle and small ruminants[35] with advanced signs of listeriosis develop metabolic acidosis as a result of salivary bicarbonate loss. Electrolyte and venous blood gas analysis helps to quantify the severity of the imbalance associated with anorexia and the salivary loss.[20,22,35,74]

Cytologic analysis of the CSF is the most useful antemortem diagnostic test to support a presumptive diagnosis of encephalitic listeriosis. Characteristic findings are an increased total protein concentration (usually >40 mg/dL) and nucleated cell count (usually >12 cells/μL), with mononuclear cells predominating.[20,22,35,36,75–77] In small ruminants, neutrophils are often observed in the CSF and, occasionally, predominate.[35] Cytologic modifications of the CSF present in cases of listeriosis may be observed in other neurologic disorders. Consequently, CSF analysis supports the presumptive diagnosis, but does not provide a definitive diagnosis.[41] Furthermore, analysis of CSF does not seem to correlate with the severity of the clinical signs or provide information on the outcome of the disease,[36] except for creatinine phosphokinase. A recent study demonstrated that creatinine phosphokinase levels in CSF had high sensitivity (100%) and specificity (100%) in predicting poor prognosis in Ossimi sheep with encephalitic listeriosis.[78] Because L monocytogenes rarely reaches the meningoventricular system, detection of the bacteria by culture or polymerase chain reaction in the CSF is frequently negative.[79]

A definitive diagnosis of encephalitic listeriosis can only be made postmortem. Pathologic confirmation of the disease is based on identification of multifocal microabscesses in the brainstem and isolation of L monocytogenes from infected brain tissue.[56] The lesions of listeric meningoencephalitis are most common in pons and medulla oblongata, but they can be located anywhere in the brainstem.[56] Neurologic structures most commonly affected include the reticular formation and cranial nerves V, VII, and XII nuclei.[80] Macroscopic lesions are limited to mild meningeal congestion and increased turbidity of the CSF.[30,51]

Characteristic microscopic lesions include multifocal asymmetrical brainstem microabscesses with areas of malacia and intense perivascular cuffing with mononuclear cells, and meningoencephalitis.[9,26,30,58,62,80,81] The microabscesses are composed predominantly of neutrophils. Other microscopic changes include multifocal gliosis, axonal swelling, and degeneration and neuronophagia.[35] Macrophages predominate in areas of extensive malacia, whereas neutrophils predominate in small microabscesses.[57,58] In animals with listeric myelitis, lesions identical to those seen in the brain are found in the spinal cord.[22,33,40] Microscopic lesions are often more acute in small ruminants than in cattle and have a more substantial neutrophilic component; likewise, microgranulomas are often observed in cattle that have encephalitic listeriosis but are seldom observed in small ruminants.[80,82]

Gram-positive rods are observed inconsistently in stained sections of brainstem from animals with encephalitic listeriosis.[57,82] The agent is only rarely isolated from CSF. For example, L monocytogenes was isolated from brain homogenates in 46% (17 of 37),[30] 45% (9 of 20),[35] and 54% (32 of 59)[82] of attempts in 3 different studies.

L monocytogenes is best recovered from refrigerated nervous tissues. Enrichment of the Listeria organisms may be accomplished by refrigerating slices of brain at 4°C (39.1°F) for 3 months while subculturing the tissues weekly.[56] A variety of media and cultural techniques have been used to promote isolation of L monocytogenes and inhibit the growth of other organisms,[4,32] but none is routinely successful at confirming a histopathologic diagnosis of listeriosis. Therefore, observation of characteristic histopathologic lesions alone is considered diagnostic for encephalitic listeriosis, even if L monocytogenes is not isolated.[15] Listeria-specific immunochemical testing of brainstem tissues is reported to be a much more efficient and rapid tool for confirmation of the histologic diagnosis of encephalitic listeriosis compared with Gram stain or bacterial culture.[5,82–86] Immunohistochemistry allows identification of listerial antigens in formalin-fixed brain tissue, even after slides have been stored for many years.[83,84]

A variety of serodiagnostic techniques exist (serum agglutination, complement fixation, ELISA) for listerial infection. Overall, serology is not routinely used for diagnosis of encephalitic listeriosis in ruminants. Detection of antibody titers against *L monocytogenes* via the agglutination test lack specificity because it cross-reacts with *Staphylococcus aureus,* enterococci, and other organisms.[87] Results using other tests have been variable, and titers generally are short lived.[88,89] Commercially available anti-listeriolysin O IgG immunoassay (ELISA) lack sensitivity and are not proven to be reliable indicators of the encephalitic form of listeriosis.[2,90,91] However, a recent study showed that the combined use of polymerase chain reaction detection of *Listeria* in milk and ELISA in the serum allowed for a rapid and effective detection of *L monocytogenes* infection in the early stage, before seroconversion, and in the later stage, even after antibiotic therapy.[92]

Last, culturing feed or bedding may be helpful in an investigation of encephalitic listeriosis.[93] A selective enrichment medium has been developed for identifying and enumerating the *Listeria* organisms in silage.[32] Using this semiquantitative enumeration method, outbreaks of listeriosis have been correlated with silage containing 1 million *Listeria* organisms and more than 1 million enterobacteria per gram of silage.[32] Furthermore, the availability of molecular diagnostic tests has enhanced the ability of scientists to investigate the role of silage feeding in encephalitic listeriosis. Polymerase chain reaction based tests recently have been developed to screen feed and environmental samples for *L monocytogenes.*[28,94] Ribotyping,[29,94,95] random amplified polymorphic DNA testing,[28] restriction enzyme analysis,[17] pulsed-field gel electrophoresis,[13] and pyrolysis mass spectrometry[96] are among the methods used in epidemiologic investigations.[15] In early reports, isolation of the same serotype of *L monocytogenes* from silage and brain was taken as presumptive evidence of an epidemiologic link.[15] Phage typing and molecular testing, however, have revealed a diversity of *L monocytogenes* strains within serotypes. Although the same strain is isolated from brain and silage in some outbreaks,[32,94] dissimilar strains are isolated in others.[94,96] During an outbreak of listeriosis, the bacterium can be isolated from the feces of animals with encephalitic listeriosis and a large percentage of normal animals.[38,43]

Treatment

Timing is everything

Treatment of encephalitic listeriosis is effective only when instituted early in the disease course. If neurologic signs have been present for several days or if recumbency or paralysis has developed, treatment is usually unrewarding.[15] Even with prompt treatment, the case fatality rate can be high, particularly in sheep and goats.[35]

Considerations

Specific treatment of encephalitic listeriosis is based on antibiotic therapy. *L monocytogenes* has been demonstrated to be sensitive in vitro to a wide range of antibiotics including penicillin, ampicillin, amoxicillin, aminoglycosides, macrolides (erythromycin), and chloramphenicol.[97] Cephalosporins are considered ineffective.[2,98] Sporadic antimicrobial resistance of clinical isolates to erythromycin, chloramphenicol, tetracycline, and streptomycin has been described.[2] Recently, an increase in antimicrobial-resistant strains of *L monocytogenes* isolated from different sources has been reported.[99,100] The proportion of isolates from a dairy environment that were resistant to penicillin, ampicillin, tetracycline, or florfenicol were 40%, 92%, 45%, and 66%, respectively.[99]

Theoretically, effective antibiotics used for the treatment of listeriosis should penetrate the intracellular space, cross the blood–brain barrier, and be bactericidal.[41] In human medicine, the recommended treatment for listeriosis is a combination of amoxicillin (or ampicillin) and an aminoglycoside (gentamicin).[98] In ruminants, few data are available to determine the best antibiotic treatment.[41] Because no antibiotics are approved for the treatment of encephalitic listeriosis in ruminants in North America, extralabel drug use requirements must be met, and banned drugs such as chloramphenicol or those with voluntary band (aminoglycosides) must be avoided.[15]

Antibiotics: options and recommended dosages

Retrospective studies of clinical cases of encephalitic listeriosis have shown no significant differences in the survival rates of cattle treated with different antibiotic regimens[22,35] and controlled trials to establish an optimum antibiotic regimen are lacking. Recommended antibiotic treatment for ruminants with encephalic listeriosis includes penicillin, ampicillin, and tetracycline. Specific recommendations for penicillin therapy include an initial dosage of 22,000 to 44,000 IU/kg, IV (potassium penicillin), 4 times daily for at least 3 to ideally 7 days and then 22,000 IU/kg, IM (procaine penicillin), twice daily for another 14 to 21 days.[41,56] However, administration of penicillin at 40,000 IU/kg twice daily IM may be sufficient when administered early in the course of the disease.[41] The recommended oxytetracycline treatment scheme requires doses as high as 10 mg/kg body weight per day for at least 5 days.[56] Both successes and failures have been reported with penicillin[21,26] and oxytetracycline.[23,27,35,51]

Clinical trials using long acting antibiotics (eg, florfenicol, tulathromycin) in the treatment of encephalitic listeriosis in ruminants are lacking. Anecdotally, one of the authors (MB) has treated 1 alpaca and 2 Boer goats with encephalitic listeriosis with florfenicol successfully.

Duration of treatment

An antibiotic treatment of long duration (2–4 weeks) is recommended to ensure a complete cure and prevent relapses.[15,101] Because of the extralabel use of the antibiotics, the high dosage used, and the long duration of treatment, withdrawal times must be extended to avoid violative residues in meat or milk.

Supportive therapy

In addition to antibiotic therapy, supportive treatment should also include oral or intravenous fluid the restore hydration and correct electrolytes and acid–base disturbances.[22,41] This measure is particularly critical, in the initial stages of listeriosis, when swallowing is difficult or impossible and antibiotic treatment has not yet taken effect.[20,101]

Administration of nonsteroidal antiinflammatory drugs has been recommended as adjunct therapy for encephalitic listeriosis.[15,41] However, their side effects (renal insufficiency and gastrointestinal ulceration) can be exacerbated in dehydrated and anorexic animals. Furthermore, their clinical efficacy is not well-described. In a recent study,[22] the use of nonsteroidal antiinflammatory drugs as adjunct therapy did not influence positively the overall survival rate of cattle with encephalitic listeriosis treated with antibiotics. It has been suggested that administration of steroidal antiinflammatory drug such as dexamethasone should be avoided owing to its inhibiting effects on cell-mediated immune responses.[102] The impact of dexamethasone treatment on the outcome of encephalitic listeriosis, however, is controversial[36] and remains to be determined.

Transfaunation,[76] feed mashes, or administration of feed orally (alfalfa meal via a stomach tube) or via a rumenostomy may contribute to maintain nutritional support during recovery. Last, adequate treatment of exposure keratitis,[15] if present, and nursing care to prevent secondary musculoskeletal injury must be provided to contribute to the overall treatment success.[101]

Prognosis

The prognosis for encephalitic listeriosis depends on the duration and severity of neurologic signs.[75] In general, it is good for cattle that are still ambulatory at the time of initial diagnosis,[15,101] but is poor for small ruminants, especially after recumbency has occurred.[22,35,101] Other than recumbency, other clinically associated poor prognostic indicators include an excitable mental state and a weak or absent menace response.[22]

In untreated cases, the fatality rate is almost 100%.[30] The survival rate in treated animals is considerably higher than in untreated patients. Reported survival rates in small ruminants and cattle with encephalitic listeriosis after treatment are 26% and 70%, respectively.[22,35] The prognosis is often guarded for advanced cases despite institution of adequate treatment.

Zoonotic Potential

Listeriosis is considered a zoonotic disease and has been reviewed recently.[7,103] Not all human cases are directly attributable to an animal source. Foodborne disease outbreaks in people have been associated with raw or improperly pasteurized milk or milk products (cheese), processed meat products, coleslaw, and contaminated raw produce including melons.[104,105] The 4b serotype of L monocytogenes most often responsible for infections in humans.[106] Cutaneous listeriosis has been observed as result of handling aborted fetuses and placentas.

All suspected material should be handled with caution. Aborted fetuses and necropsy of septicemic animals present the greatest hazard. In cases with encephalitis, L monocytogenes is usually confined to the brain and presents little risk of transmission unless the brain is removed. Protective personal equipment should be worn when handling or during necropsy of ruminants with listeriosis.

Prevention

Because L monocytogenes is widely distributed in the environment, prevention of encephalitic listeriosis is based on reducing the exposure to L monocytogenes and minimizing stressful conditions that may increase susceptibility to infection. Biosecurity and hygiene practices are important for reducing the risk of introduction and perpetuation of L monocytogenes on farms.[38] The risk of encephalitic listeriosis can be decreased in ruminants by feeding good quality silage with adequate anaerobic conditions and a low pH.[71] A heavy inoculation of organisms from soil or feces should be avoided and, in exceptional circumstances, it has been recommended that pastures identified for making silage be kept free of grazing animals during the spring.[2] Spoiled or moldy silage should be avoided, as well as silage from the superficial few inches exposed to air. Any leftover silage should be removed after feeding. Rotten vegetation should be discarded, and cattle should be fenced off from contaminated areas. Equipment used to handle abnormal silage or fecal matter should be thoroughly cleaned before handling feed to prevent cross-contamination.[15] Steps should be taken to avoid overcrowding of animals and minimize weather- and housing-related stressors. Culturing feed, bedding, soil, and water sources may be helpful in an outbreak investigation of encephalitic listeriosis.[49,93] New animals added to the herd should be quarantined, and animals with clinical listeriosis isolated.

Numerous vaccines of attenuated or killed *L monocytogenes* have been developed, some of which have resulted in a reduction in the incidence or severity of encephalitic listeriosis under natural or experimental conditions compared with unvaccinated controls.[16,88,107–109] Although these vaccines reduce the incidence of listeriosis in vaccinated flocks, they are not currently available in the United States.[15,56,71]

Summary

In ruminants, encephalitic listeriosis should be suspected when depression and multiple cranial nerve deficits are observed. Ascending infection of the causative agent, *L monocytogenes* from the terminal roots of the trigeminal nerve, from breaches in the oral mucous membranes to the brainstem, is the most accepted pathogenesis. The disease is typically sporadic, but may affect several animals in a herd over a short period of time.

Presumptive antemortem diagnosis is made on the basis of neurologic signs and by observing increases in protein concentration and mononuclear cells in CSF. Definitive diagnosis of encephalitic listeriosis at necropsy is made by detecting characteristic histopathologic lesions, including microabscesses, multifocal gliosis, and mononuclear perivascular cuffing in the brainstem and isolating the causative agent from infected brain tissue. Immunohistochemistry is used to detect *L monocytogenes* antigens in formalin-fixed brain tissue and is more sensitive than bacteriologic culture.

Treatment involves a prolonged course of parenteral antibiotic therapy (penicillin, ampicillin, or oxytetracycline) and is more successful in cattle than in sheep and goats. Treatment should be initiated early and is seldom effective after animals are recumbent.

Outbreaks of encephalitic listeriosis usually occur in winter and are often attributed to consumption of poorly fermented silage; however, encephalitic listeriosis can develop on any diet at any time of the year. Because fecal shedding by clinically healthy ruminants is the most likely source of *L monocytogenes*, efforts should be made to avoid fecal contamination of feed.[15]

OTITIS MEDIA/INTERNA

Otitis externa, OM, and otitis interna are associated with inflammation of the external ear, middle ear, and inner ear, respectively. OM and OMI have been reported in all domestic food animal species worldwide. In veterinary medicine, OM is by far the most common cause of facial nerve paralysis.[110]

Etiology

A wide variety of bacteria, mites, and nematodes have been isolated from the otic discharge or tympanic bullae of food animal species with OMI. In ruminants (cattle, sheep, goats, camelids), most cases are attributed to bacterial infection. Respiratory tract pathogens including *H somni*,[111,112] *Mannheimia haemolytica*,[113,114] *Mycoplasma bovis*,[115–119] and *Pasteurella multocida*[113,114,120] are often isolated, as is *Trueperella pyogenes* (formerly *Arcanobacterium pyogenes*)[113,114] in more chronic cases.

M bovis, either alone or in association with other bacteria, is becoming increasingly recognized as the main etiologic agent of OMI in dairy calves.[115–119,121,122] Although the relative prevalence of *Mycoplasma* spp.-associated OMI seems to be increased, the true prevalence and importance of the disease is not well-characterized. Confounding factors include difficulty to culture *Mycoplasma* spp. and the fact that both pathogenic and nonpathogenic *Mycoplasma* spp. can be harbored in the external ear canals of apparently healthy animals.[113,123,124]

Corynebacterium pseudotuberculosis,[120,125] *L monocytogenes*,[24] coliforms,[126] *Streptococcus* spp, *Staphylococcus* spp,[122] and *Pseudomonas aeruginosa*[122,127] have also been isolated sporadically from cattle, sheep, goats, and camelids with OMI, alone or in conjunction with the aforementioned bacteria. Mixed bacterial populations are not uncommon,[113,114,120,122,126,128] and bacteria may be found in conjunction with parasites.[124,129,130]

In tropical and subtropical areas, parasitic otitis externa is a major problem in cattle. It can reach the middle ear through a ruptured tympanic membrane and extend to the inner ear, resulting in OMI.[15,121] The nematode parasite *Rhabditis bovis* is an important cause of bovine otitis in areas such South Africa and South America during warm and humid weather.[129,131,132] Fortunately, this condition does not exist in North America.[15] In more temperate regions such as North America, the ear mites associated with otitis are *Raillietia auris* (cattle),[133] *Raillietia caprae* (goats), and *Psoroptes cuniculi* (goats).[124,134] However, these parasites can be found in the external ear canals of many apparently healthy animals.[135,136]

In pigs, *Streptococcus* spp., particularly *Streptococcus suis*, is by far the most common cause of clinical and subclinical OMI.[137] Other bacterial pathogens incriminated in this species include *P multocida*, *Actinobacillus pleuropneumonia*, *T pyogenes*, *Haemophilus* spp., *Mycoplasma hyopneumonia*,[138,139] and *Mycoplasma hyorhinitis*.[140]

Epidemiology

OMI is a common disease in ruminants. Sporadic cases,[112] as well as outbreaks,[113] have been described. All ages and sexes may be affected, but young animals seem to be particularly susceptible, especially young livestock in the preweaning and postweaning periods, as are yearlings.[119,120] Reportedly, beef calves are more often affected, although the incidence of OMI seems to be increasing among dairy calves. This increase in dairy production animals is thought to be owing to an increasing rate of *M bovis* infections.[15,116–118,141] Peak incidence of clinical *M bovis*–induced OM in dairy calves occurs at 2 to 8 weeks of age.[113,117] Except for parasite-induced otitis in subtropical and tropical regions,[124,129,132,133] bacterial OMI seems to be uncommon to rare in adult ruminants with only a limited number of cases reported.[142]

The incidence of OMI is increased in the winter months or during inclement weather.[111,113,115,117,118,122] The true prevalence of OMI in ruminants is unknown and likely underestimated. Confounding factors include poor sensitivity or delay in making a presumptive clinical diagnosis, overall poor sensitivity of diagnostic tests available to primary care veterinarians, and difficulty in accessing the auditory system at necropsy for definitive diagnosis.[15,126] Clinical diagnosis may be missed early in the disease process because the condition can remain subclinical. It often becomes chronic by the time neurologic deficits are obvious.[115,116]

In young intensively reared cattle and sheep, morbidity ranges from 20% to 100% during outbreaks.[112–114,120,121,126] In feedlot cattle, herd morbidity estimates range from 1% to 20%.[111,120] In dairy cattle, morbidity estimates range from 1% to as high as 80% in individually housed calves.[128,143] Sporadic individual cases can occur in goats,[125,134] camelids,[24,144,145] and pigs.[137]

Risk Factors

Bottle feeding and feeding contaminated colostrum or milk have been identified as risk factors for the development of OM in lambs[146] and dairy calves.[117] Maunsell and colleagues[147] recently demonstrated that oral inoculation of young calves with *M bovis*-contaminated milk resulted in an ascending infection of the Eustachian (auditory) tubes and development of OM similar to that found in natural disease. They concluded that the upper respiratory tract, in particular the pharyngeal tonsils, represent the major site of colonization by *M bovis* after oral inoculation. This pattern of colonization of the Eustachian tube and development of eustachitis preceding OM is consistent with *Mycoplasma hyorhinis* infection in pigs.[140]

However, the main risk factor associated with the development of OM is the presence of a coincidental respiratory infection. Many studies document bacterial OM in conjunction with or after respiratory disease,[114,115,117,118,120,122,143,146] with the same causative pathogens isolated.[15]

In tropical and subtropical regions, the incidence of parasitic otitis is greatest during the rainy season, primarily owing to the high environmental temperatures and relative humidity. Bos indicus cattle with long, pendant, and gutter-shaped ear pinna or cattle breeds with larger horns seem to be at increased risk for parasitic otitis.[121,132] In addition, cattle dipped regularly in acaricide-containing tank for the control of tickborne disease such as East coast fever experience a higher incidence of otitis (70%) caused by nematode *R bovis* compared with those sprayed by the same acaricide (5%).[131] Reportedly, viable nematodes have been recovered from 0.25% toxaphene dip wash tanks.[131]

Pathogenesis

OM may result from the extension of an otitis externa, colonization of the middle ear from the Eustachian tube, or hematogenous spread. In tropical and subtropical areas, nematode parasites represent the most common cause of otitis externa. Parasites and accompanying purulent and necrotic debris present in the external ear progress into the middle ear compartment through a damaged or ruptured tympanic membrane.[15,121,129,133–135] Ascending infection of the Eustachian tube is the primary route by which bacterial pathogens enter the middle ear. Pathogenic bacteria frequently colonize the nasopharynx and tonsils[147] and gain access to the Eustachian tube (which extends from the nasopharynx to the middle ear) via the pharyngeal ostium.[120,126,148] This is a logical route of infection for OM in calves fed contaminated milk or colostrum,[117] in bottle fed lambs,[146] and in animals with concurrent respiratory infections.[115,118,120,146] Last, the pathogens can also reach the middle ear by hematogenous spread, but this is thought to occur rarely because most animals with OM have no signs of bacteremia.[15] Although the importance of hematogenous spread in the development of OM is likely minimal, OM have been reported in animals with an intact tympanic membrane and no evidence of respiratory disease.[115]

Infection of the middle ear may remain localized or may spread to other parts of the ear. Accumulation of exudate and increased pressure in the middle ear compartment result in rupture of the tympanic membrane, which allows extension of infection to the external ear with subsequent development of otic discharge.[15] Alternatively, infection of the inner ear (otitis interna, labyrinthitis) can develop and, if left untreated, can progress to osteomyelitis and extend into the calvarium. Invasion of the infection through the dura mater often leads to brain abscessation or to disseminated meningitis.[112,114] OMI is usually unilateral, but at least 25% of cases had bilateral involvement in several reports.[120,126,143,146,148]

Clinical Signs

Clinical signs associated with otitis externa owing to mites *R auris*, *R caprae*, or *P cuniculi*, include head shaking, ear rubbing or scratching, otorrhea, inflammation (erythema, scabs, ulcerations), cellulitis of the external ear canal, and aural hematoma.[124,133,134] Foul smelling blood-tinged to dark-brown otic discharge, sloughing of the affected ear pinna, and cachexia have also been described in cattle with chronic *R bovis*-associated otitis externa in tropical and subtropical regions.[129,131] The parasites and associated inflammatory response damage the tympanic membrane, which in some cases allows invasion of the middle ear by mites, nematodes, or bacteria.[121,124,134]

Clinical signs associated with OMI are attributable to dysfunction of cranial nerves VII (facial) and VIII (vestibulocochlear). Because of the anatomic location of these nerves, lesions of the facial nerve develop with infection of the middle ear, whereas lesions of the vestibulocochlear nerve appear with extension of the infection into the inner ear.[41,110,138]

Lesions of the facial nerve produce ear droop (unilateral or bilateral) and palpebral ptosis (**Fig. 2**). Exposure keratitis and epiphora may develop secondary to the paresis or paralysis of the eyelid. Ipsilateral lip droop may also be evident. Collapse of the ipsilateral nostril and deviation of the upper lip to the opposite side can be seen in small ruminants and camelids. In some cases, purulent aural discharge is observed after rupture of the tympanic membrane.[113,119,120,122] It is reported to develop 2 to 3 days after appearance of clinical signs.[113,128] Ear pain evidenced by head shaking and scratching or rubbing ears can be observed in calves.[115,117,141,149] Matting of hair around the base of the ear and erythema of the pinna may be seen,[113,114,119] and secondary myiasis may occur.[144] Concurrent clinical signs of pneumonia are frequently observed in calves with OM.[115–118,149] Animals with uncomplicated OM are alert and have a good appetite. However, they become febrile and anorexic as the disease progresses. Severely affected calves may also maintain a good suckle reflex until death.[15]

Otitis interna is a common sequela to OM, and affected animals exhibit varying degrees of peripheral (unilateral or bilateral) vestibular dysfunction.[110] Patients with unilateral otitis interna show head tilt (see **Fig. 2**) and vestibular ataxia characterized by leaning, falling, or rolling toward the side of the lesion,[117,118,141,149] which worsens after blindfolding. In animals with bilateral otitis interna, no postural asymmetry is noted.

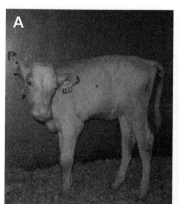
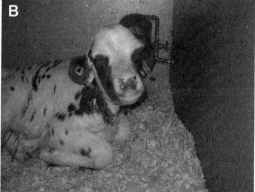

Fig. 2. (*A*) Two-month-old Ayrshire heifer calf with unilateral otitis media/interna. The left-sided head tilt, ear droop, and ptosis indicates involvement of the left facial and vestibulo-cochlear nerve (cranial nerves VII and VIII, respectively). (*B*) One-month-old Ayrshire heifer calf with bilateral otitis media and concurrent pneumonia. Note the bilateral ear droop and ptosis. (*Courtesy of* David Francoz, DVM, MSc, Faculté de médecine vétérinaire, Université de Montréal, Saint-Hyacinthe, Québec, Canada.)

Balance is lost to either side, resulting in the patient assuming a crouched posture closer to the ground surface and a slow and cautious ambulation to prevent falling.[110] In these cases, the presence of wide head excursions to either side and to the same degree is often characteristic.[110] Horizontal nystagmus ipsilateral to the head tilt and body deviation may be present in cases of otitis interna with central vestibular lesions.[110] Classification of severity of clinical and neurologic findings in calves with OM and OMI via a scoring system has been described recently.[122]

Other clinical signs that have been associated recently with *M bovis* OMI in calves include spontaneous regurgitation of milk or rumen fluid, loss of pharyngeal tone, dorsal displacement of the soft palate, and dysphagia, indicative of glossopharyngeal nerve dysfunction with or without vagal nerve dysfunction.[116,141,150] Whether these nerves are affected by inflammation associated with meningitis or secondary to inflammation at the sites where the nerves pass over the tympanic bullae is unknown.[141]

In advanced cases of otitis interna, extension of infection to the meninges results in depression, ataxia, opisthotonos, seizure or sudden death with no preceding clinical signs.[112,115,117,118,141]

Diagnosis

A presumptive diagnosis of OMI in a live animal can be made on the basis of history, physical examination, and, most important, clinical evidence of facial and/or vestibulocochlear nerve disease. The presumptive clinical diagnosis can be confirmed by otoscopic examination, deep ear swabs, and various diagnostic imaging techniques.[115,141,151,152]

Ear swab

When otorrhea is present, deep ear swab samples should be collected, examined microscopically for parasites, and submitted both for aerobic bacterial and *Mycoplasma spp.* culture.[119] Mites and nematodes can reside deep in the ear canal close to the tympanic membrane, making them difficult to detect even with deep swabbing.[121] In cattle, irrigation of the external ear canal is a more sensitive diagnostic technique compared with swabbing the affected ear in case of mite infestation.[153]

Detection of a considerable number of mites[135] or nematodes[129] in the external ear canal or heavy growth of a pure culture of a bacterial organism from otic discharge coupled with suggestive clinical signs supports a diagnosis of OM, but could also be incidental. Some pathogens reported to induce OM such as *R auris* (previously described as 1 mm white to cream color sphere/ovoid body with dark brown legs),[133,135] *R caprae*, and *P cuniculi*,[124,134] or *Mycoplasma* spp.[136,154] may be isolated from the external ear of apparently healthy ruminants. Specific bacterial culture, molecular or immunologic diagnostic techniques for *M bovis*, sample collection, and sample handling and transport have been reviewed previously.[150]

Visualizing the tympanic membrane

Visualization of a hyperemic and bulging or ruptured tympanic membrane is suggestive and indicative of OM, respectively.[113] However, some animals, particularly sheep[126,146] and milk-fed calves,[117,148] may have intact tympanic membranes. Otoscopic visualization of the tympanic membrane in ruminants is hampered by the length of the ear canal and by copious or tenacious exudate in the ear.[122] In camelids, otoscopic examination of the tympanic membrane is impossible owing to the sigmoid shape of the bony ear canal.[144] Endoscopic examination has facilitated visualization of the tympanic membrane in some cases.[122] Overall, visualization of the tympanic membranes is neither very sensitive nor specific. In a recent study, agreement between otoscopy and neurologic deficits present in calves with OM or OMI was 77%.[122]

Diagnostic imaging
Radiographic images of the tympanic bulla of calves have been reported to be useful for the diagnosis of OMI.[114] Evaluation of the tympanic bulla is best achieved with a lateral oblique view.[41] The inability to open ruminant mouths widely inhibits the use of open-mouth projections to compare the 2 tympanic bullae. In addition, the presence of trabeculations within the tympanic bulla in cattle decreases the contrast between the air-filled bulla and bone. The normal trabeculations produce increased opacity within the bulla making radiographic assessment difficult, which may lead to a false-positive diagnosis of OMI.[151] In 1 retrospective study involving 29 dairy calves with this disorder,[116] radiographic abnormalities of affected tympanic bullae included increased opacity, size and thickening of the osseous bulla, lysis of the trabeculae and of the wall, and irregularity of the hyoid bone. Overall, radiographs of the tympanic bulla should be considered as a specific but not sensitive diagnostic tool.[151] In camelids, injection of contrast media into the ear may facilitate visualization of the ear canal and allow assessment of tympanic membrane integrity.[144]

Computed tomography (CT) imaging may provide the best detail for both the osseous and soft tissue changes that occur in cases of OMI.[110] However, such procedures are limited to referral centers and valuable animals. CT imaging has been reported for the diagnosis of OMI in calves[141] and other ruminant species including camelids[145,155] and a North American bison.[156] The most frequent CT abnormality associated with a diagnosis of OM is increased soft tissue opacity within the tympanic bulla and osteolysis of the trabeculae.[151] CT is considered the gold standard antemortem diagnostic modality in calves because it allows for the diagnosis of clinical and subclinical cases of OM and OMI.[151]

Recently, ultrasound imaging of the tympanic bulla has been investigated as a diagnostic tool for diagnosis of clinical and subclinical OMI in young calves.[116,152] This imaging modality can be useful to define the extent of damage to the tympanic bulla, and evaluate the progression of lesions over time.[116] In a study involving 40 veal calves at 3 to 7 weeks of age, ultrasound imaging of both tympanic bullae was used in the diagnosis of OM and compared with histopathologic findings on postmortem examination.[152] In this study, 45 of the 80 tympanic bullae (56%) were affected by OM. The sensitivity and specificity of ultrasound imaging of tympanic bullae for the diagnosis of clinical and subclinical OM ranged from 32% to 63% and 84% to 100%, respectively.[152] The same group of researchers has since published specific guidelines to standardize and ease the learning curve of this ultrasound technique.[157] Briefly, a high-frequency (7.5–10 MHz), short linear (38 mm) probe is recommended.[157]

Other antemortem diagnostics
In most cases of OM or OMI, complete blood count and serum biochemistry profile are of little diagnostic value. Hematology and serum biochemistry findings can be unremarkable[122] or show evidence of an inflammatory leukogram (neutrophilia, monocytosis) with an increase in fibrinogen.[115] When pneumonia is associated with OMI, the same etiologic agent may be responsible for both diseases.[115] Consequently, culture of a transtracheal lavage may be useful to identify the pathogens and recommend appropriate antimicrobial treatment.

OMI can extend to the cranial cavity through osteomyelitis of the petrous part of the temporal bone.[110] Unless complicated by meningitis, CSF analysis is normal in cases of OMI.[115] However, a mononuclear pleocytosis can be present on CSF analysis with and without osteolysis on radiographs.[116] In such cases, it has been postulated that the migration of the inflammation or infection could occur along the facial nerve through the internal acoustic meatus to reach the medulla. Pleocytosis may then be detected in the CSF, not associated with an abscess or diffuse meningitis.[77]

Postmortem diagnosis

A definitive diagnosis of OM or OMI can be confirmed ultimately on postmortem examination.[15] Several techniques to approach the middle and inner ear have been described.[120,126,158] Gross lesions depend on the extent and duration of infection and include erythema and swelling of the tympanic membrane; erythema, edema, or thickening of the mucosa of the auditory system; exudate or caseous material in the tympanic cavity; rupture of the tympanic membrane with accumulation of exudate in external ear canal; destruction or sclerosis of bony structures in and around the ear; and replacement of bony structures by granulation tissue.[118,120,126,127,147,149] Samples must be decalcified for histologic examination.[117] Histopathologic findings include fibrinosuppurative inflammation in the tympanic cavities, in the surrounding bone, and in other auditory structures; osteolysis and/or remodeling of the adjacent bone; and perineural inflammation of the facial or vestibulocochlear nerves.[24,117,118,141,149] Inflammation may extend into the Eustachian tubes.[118,144,146]

Finding concurrent pneumonia, especially in calves, is common.[118,149] In 1 study, concurrent pneumonia occurred in 47 cases (77%), and *Mycoplasma* spp. was isolated from the lungs of 30 of those cases.[118] Chronic cases may show cachexia with serous atrophy of perirenal and pericardial fat.[117] With meningitis, the CSF may be cloudy and the meninges covered with fibrinopurulent exudate.[112,118,159]

Treatment

Specific treatment of OM depends on the etiologic agent. If left untreated, it can progress to otitis interna and meningitis.[114]

Parasitic otitis

Topical drugs (ethyl alcohol; ethyl ester solution (1:1 ratio (v/v)) containing 2% copper sulfate)[121] and acaricide mixtures (rotenone and fenthion)[134] have been used for the treatment of parasitic otitis externa with varying degree of success.[129] Overall, reinfection is common and frequent treatment is vital. In animals with ruptured tympanic membranes, topical instillation of acaricide is contraindicated.[121] In the latter cases, cleaning and flushing of the external ear canal in conjunction with parenteral administration of ivermectin is recommended.[15,121,153] Ivermectin, when given subcutaneously at a dosage of 10 mg/50 kg of body weight, was found to be greater than 95% effective in the treatment of *Railletia* spp.–associated otitis in cattle.[160] Adjunct antibiotic therapy is often warranted,[121] especially in cases developing secondary bacterial OM or OMI.

Bacterial otitis media/interna

Treatment of OMI is based on the institution of antibiotic therapy, which must be effective against the most frequently isolated pathogens and diffuse into the middle and the inner ear.[41] There are no antibiotics approved for the treatment of OMI in ruminants; therefore, extralabel drug use requirements must be observed.[15] Antibiotic treatment is best selected on the basis of culture results, but because mixed bacterial infections are common, broad-spectrum antibiotic therapy is appropriate.[15] Concurrent conditions such as pneumonia (eg, *Mycoplasma* spp.) also must be treated appropriately.

Antibiotics that could be used to treat *Mycoplasma* infections in cattle are tetracycline, spectinomycin, tylosin, tilmicosin, florfenicol, fluoroquinolones such as enrofloxacin,[41,150] tulathromycin,[122] and gamithromycin. In the United States, tulathromycin

(Draxxin, Zoetis, Kalamazoo, MI), gamithromycin (Gamithromycin, Zactran, Merial, Duluth, GA), enrofloxaxin (Baytril 100, Bayer HealthCare LLC, Animal Health Division, Shawnee Mission, KS), and florfenicol (Nuflor Gold Antimicrobial, Merck Animal Health/Intervet, Summit, NJ) are the only 4 drugs approved for the treatment of *M bovis*-associated bovine respiratory disease in beef and nonlactating dairy cattle, all as single-dose therapy. Recent evidence suggests that antimicrobial resistance to antibiotics traditionally used for treatment of *Mycoplasma* infections is increasing in field isolates of *M bovis* in North America.[161,162] North American isolates show widespread resistance to tetracyclines and tilmicosin.

There are very few clinical trials evaluating the efficacy of antibiotics available for treatment of OMI in ruminants. Most have been done in calves with *Mycoplasma* spp. as the primary underlying etiology of the disease.[113,115,122] Successful treatment of OMI in dairy calves has been reported with enrofloxacin[113,115] however this antibiotic is only approved by the US Food and Drug Administration for the treatment of respiratory disease in beef cattle, nonlactating dairy cattle and swine and extralabel use of this drug is prohibited. In a recent prospective study, Bertone and colleagues[122] evaluated the effectiveness of tulathromycin, oxytetracycline (injectable then oral) and carprofen as a therapeutic standardized protocol for acute onset of OM and OMI in 22 veal calves primarily owing to *M bovis* (alone or in combination with other bacteria in 89% of affected ears). Total treatment time was 14 days. Significant improvement of clinical and neurologic scores was observed in 20 of 22 calves (90%) and a full recovery in only 1 of the 22 (5%). No worsening of clinical conditions was observed or further treatments required at the 1-month follow-up.

The optimal therapy regimen and associated duration for OM and OMI in cattle and other ruminants remains to be determined. The duration of the treatment is influenced by the chronicity of the disease, as well as the implicated pathogens. Proposed duration of treatment ranges from 5 days to several weeks[113,115,122,128] Acute disease has been reported to be treated successfully with antibiotics, whereas such treatment for chronic disease may not be successful despite an extended duration of antibiotic therapy.[115,117,120,141,163] In feedlots, chronic otitis in older animals was suspected to be a recurrence of an OM contracted as calves.[120]

Adjunct therapy

Irrigation of the middle ear after the tympanic membrane has ruptured has been recommended for treatment of undifferentiated OM in calves.[15,114,134] Many irrigation solutions have been used, with isotonic saline being the most common, but none has been shown definitively to be superior.[15,114]

Puncture of the tympanic membrane (myringotomy) followed by insertion of tympanostomy tubes is commonly used in the treatment of children with chronic or recurrent OM,[164] and some veterinarians have promoted blind myringotomy using a sharp object such as a knitting needle in the treatment of OM in calves.[165] In a recent study using calf cadavers, investigators reported that blind insertion of a 3.5-mm diameter straight knitting needle approximately 3 cm into the ear canal to perforate the tympanic membrane was anatomically feasible.[166] To the best of the authors' knowledge, studies on the risks and efficacy of this procedure in clinical cases have not been published. The potential benefit of myringotomy is the relief of pain and pressure caused by the buildup of exudate in the middle ear, as well as access to the middle ear for irrigation. Whether the procedure might provide relief for calves that have the thick, caseous exudate characteristic of chronic *M bovis* OM is not clear.

Surgical treatment such as total or subtotal ear canal ablation with tympanic bulla osteotomy combined with short- or long-term systemic antibiotic therapy has been reported to be successful in calves,[141] goats,[134] alpacas,[155] and a bison[156] with chronic OMI. In contrast, a surgical approach was unsuccessful in a llama.[144] Because of the cost and complexity associated with this procedure, as well as the requirement for general anesthesia, its application is probably limited to refractory cases of OM or OMI in valuable animals without concurrent respiratory disease.

The use of regional long-term antibiotic therapy in the treatment of chronic OM is not well-documented. Only 1 report described placement of cefazolin-impregnated poly-methylmethacrylate beads within the affected tympanic bullae of a bison after total ear canal ablation and bulla curettage.[156] Six months after surgery, the animal had no recurrent signs of OM.

Although nonsteroidal anti-inflammatory drugs have not been evaluated specifically for the treatment of OMI, there is a logical basis for their use, because the inflammatory response may contribute significantly to the pathology of the disease. Other nonspecific supportive therapy, including oral or intravenous fluids, nutritional support, treatment of corneal ulceration, and protection from self-inflicted injury, may be indicated.[15,141]

Prognosis

The prognosis for OM or OMI depends on the chronicity of the disease and the etiologic agent involved. The outcome of treatment is variable and seems to be better in calves than yearling cattle or small ruminants.[15,120] Treatment in the acute stages has been effective,[122] although poor response to therapy has been related to chronicity or development of complications.[15,111,113–115,120,145,147] Chronic cases usually require extended antibiotic therapy owing to involvement of the surrounding bone. They can also become refractory to treatment.[15,150] Case fatality rates range from 0% to 100%.[15] The overall prognosis for OMI ranges from guarded[117] to good.[115] Calves with chronic OMI receiving long-term antimicrobial therapy tend to adapt and thrive despite the persistence of neurologic signs.[115,116,122,167]

Economic Losses

In tropical and subtropical regions, R bovis-associated otitis in cattle causes major economic losses as a result of weight loss, decreased milk production, infertility, death, and condemnation of heads and carcasses at slaughter.[121,131] In calves and yearlings with OM, economic losses are attributed to decreased growth/poor weight gain, extensive antibiotic therapy and associated labor, and from condemnation of heads and carcasses at rendering facilities.[120]

In a recent prospective cohort study, veal calves with respiratory disease were found to be 2.2 and 2.4 times more likely to develop arthritis and otitis, respectively.[167] In this study, OM was not associated with decreased growth; however, calves showing clinical signs were treated with antibiotics. And although none of the calves died from otitis only, otitis did increase the mortality risk (hazard ratio, 7.0).

Prevention

Control measures and treatment for parasitic otitis in tropical and subtropical regions are not yet standardized and their efficacy is not consistent in the literature.[121] The most relevant preventative measures for R bovis-associated otitis externa in cattle include but are not limited to appropriate fly control, frequent removal and proper disposal of organic material, use of an acaricide spray instead of a dip tank,[131] dehorning of calves, and monitoring and control of infestations of older animals with larger horns.[121] Ear mite infestation can be controlled by use of injectable ivermectin, with repeated dosing at 2- to 3-week intervals required to eradicate the mites.[15] Overall, bovine parasitic otitis should be considered as a herd infection requiring herd, rather than individual, treatment.[129]

At-risk animals such as cattle entering the feedlot, calves fed waste milk, and animals with respiratory disease should be monitored for signs of OM or OMI and treated promptly.[15] Measures should be taken to minimize nutritional and environmental stress and to prevent respiratory disease because these seem to be predisposing factors.[114,115,117,118,120,122,143,146] In dairy herds with *Mycoplasma* spp. mastitis, unpasteurized bulk tank, waste milk, or colostrum should not be fed to calves or should be appropriately pasteurized before feeding.[117] *M bovis* is killed by pasteurization at 65°C for 2 minutes.[168] Calves with concurrent *Mycoplasma* pneumonia should be isolated from others and cared for separately.[150] More specific control measures for *Mycoplasma* infection in calves have been described previously.[150]

Summary

OMI occurs sporadically in cattle, sheep, goats, camelids, and pigs. A variety of bacteria, including *Mycoplasma* spp, and parasites (mites in North America), have been implicated. Young animals seem to be particularly susceptible, especially young livestock in the preweaning and postweaning period, as in yearlings. The incidence of OMI is increased in the winter months or during inclement weather. Most cases seem to result from ascending infection through the Eustachian tube or extension of infection from the external ear. Respiratory tract infection and feeding of infected milk or colostrum seem to be risk factors for OMI, as does severe ear mite or nematode infestation.[15] Clinical signs of facial nerve (cranial nerve VII) damage, such as ear droop and ptosis, are associated with OM, whereas signs of vestibulocochlear nerve (cranial nerve VIII) damage, such as head tilt, leaning, falling, circling, and horizontal nystagmus, indicate otitis interna.[15] Cattle, goats, and camelids with OMI frequently have purulent otorrhea, but this is rare in sheep. The presumptive diagnosis is based on clinical and neurologic signs, deep ear swab, and otoscopic examination. Ultrasound imaging of the tympanic bullae in calves up to 10 weeks old, skull radiographs, CT imaging (gold standard) and, ultimately, postmortem examination can be used to confirm the clinical diagnosis.

The prognosis is variable and treatment involves early recognition and prompt administration of appropriate antibiotics or anthelmintics; irrigation of the ear canal and supportive measures may be required in some cases.[15] Chronic cases usually require extended antibiotic therapy and may benefit from surgical treatment. However, those cases as well as animals with signs of meningitis secondary to otitis interna have a poor prognosis for recovery.

PITUITARY ABSCESS SYNDROME

Pituitary abscess syndrome is an uncommon neurologic disease typically responsible for progressive signs of cerebral and brainstem dysfunction. The syndrome has been reported in cattle,[72,169–171] goats,[81,172] sheep,[173] horses,[174] and humans.[175] The condition generally occurs secondary to other septic processes in variable locations throughout the body. Pituitary abscess syndrome is an important differential diagnosis for other central nervous system disorders such as encephalitic listeriosis, OMI, and rabies. Pituitary abscess syndrome has been reviewed previously.[15]

Etiology

The most common bacterial species isolated from cases of pituitary abscess syndrome is *T pyogenes*.[72,81,169,173] Other bacterial species commonly isolated include

Staphylococcus sp., *Streptococcus* sp., *Fusobacterium necrophorum*, and *C pseudo-tuberculosis*.[72,81,176] *Mycoplasma arginini* was isolated from a single goat with a pituitary abscess.[172]

Pathogenesis

Pituitary abscess syndrome generally occurs secondary to other septic processes and is thought to result from hematogenous spread of bacteria in the rete mirabile[15] (**Fig. 3**), a complex network of intertwined blood vessels surrounding the pituitary gland of ruminants and other species.[177] In a retrospective study of 20 cases of pituitary abscess, Perdrizet and Dinsmore[72] found sites of chronic infection separate from the pituitary gland in 11 of 20 cases. Sites of infection identified by clinical history included tooth abscess, mastitis, bronchopneumonia, and sinusitis. Details of other sites of infection identified at necropsy were not provided. Seven of the lesions were cultured and 5 contained the same bacteria as found in the pituitary abscess. Although hematogenous spread of bacteria is thought to be the most common route by which bacteria gain access to the pituitary gland, other routes of infections have been reported. Müller and colleagues[170] reported the occurrence of pituitary abscess syndrome in a Simmental heifer secondary to postdehorning sinusitis and osteomyelitis of the sphenoid bone. Bacterial migration along lymphatics has also been hypothesized as an alternate route by which bacteria may gain access to the pituitary gland.[169]

Risk Factors

Several authors have described the occurrence of pituitary abscess syndrome after the use of nose flaps for weaning calves[169,176,178] or the placement of nose rings.[179] In 1 report, weaning flaps were left in for 7 days with neurologic abnormalities developing 6 to 7 days after flap removal.[176] In another report, flaps were in place for 3 to 7 days with clinical signs occurring 12 to 60 days after placement of the flaps.[169]

Clinical Signs

The clinical signs of pituitary abscess syndrome are variable and nonspecific, but typically include signs of cerebral and brainstem dysfunction. The most common sign of cerebral dysfunction is depression (**Fig. 4**).[72,169,170] Recumbency, opisthotonus and

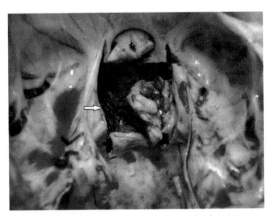

Fig. 3. Normal appearance of the rete mirabile (*arrow*) of a bovine on postmortem examination. The rete mirabile is a complex network of intertwined blood vessels surrounding the pituitary gland of ruminants and other species.

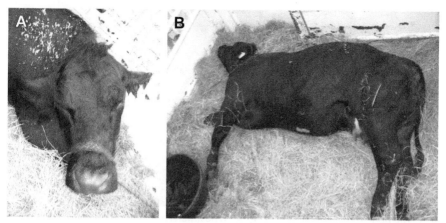

Fig. 4. (*A*) Five-year-old Angus cow with pituitary abscess syndrome. Note the severe mental depression. (*B*) The same cow as in (*A*). The cow is now comatose and remains laterally recumbent.

convulsions may be seen in terminal stages of the disease.[72,169,179] Signs of brainstem dysfunction and accompanying cranial nerve deficits are typically asymmetrical and include facial paralysis, dysphagia, jaw and tongue hypotonia, decreased facial sensation, and head tilt.[72,169,176] Abnormalities found on neuroophthalmologic examination include blindness, abnormal pupillary light reflexes, strabismus, and nystagmus.[72,169–171,173] Exophthalmos has been reported[169,171,176,179] and is thought to occur owing to extension of inflammation into the orbit.

Bradycardia is reported to occur in up to 50% of cases and is thought to be owing to compression of the hypothalamus.[72] Reported clinical signs related to other body systems other than bradycardia are variable and nonspecific.

Diagnosis

A presumptive diagnosis of pituitary abscess syndrome is typically based on characteristic clinical and neurologic signs. Identification of a site of chronic infection distant from the central nervous system in an animal with consistent neurologic signs may increase the likelihood of pituitary abscess syndrome. Changes in complete blood count and serum biochemistry are variable and inconsistent. Reported changes are consistent with infection or inflammation and include changes in white blood cell count (primarily mature neutrophilia), increased serum protein levels, and increases in fibrinogen.[72,170]

Reported changes in CSF are also variable. Perdrizet and Dinsmore[72] reported consistently elevated protein levels and mild to marked pleocytosis in 5 animals in which CSF analysis was performed. In a more recent report, Stokol and colleagues[77] found no difference in CSF findings in cattle with pituitary abscess, vertebral body abscess, or spinal epidural abscess with protein concentrations and cell counts ranging from normal to markedly elevated. Pleocytosis has been reported to be primarily neutrophilic[72] or primarily mononuclear.[77]

Although advanced diagnostic imaging such as CT or MRI could potentially be useful in the diagnosis of pituitary abscess syndrome, published reports are lacking. A single report describes the use of CT to diagnose a cerebral abscess (not involving the pituitary gland) in a calf.[180]

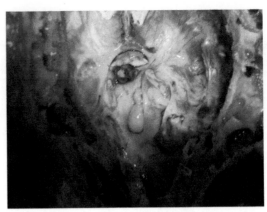

Fig. 5. The brain of the cow shown in **Fig. 4** on postmortem. Note the purulent discharge in the area of the pituitary gland.

The measurement of pituitary hormone levels may potentially be useful in the diagnosis of pituitary dysfunction. Dabak and colleagues[173] described a single case of confirmed pituitary abscess in sheep in which thyroid stimulating hormone, follicle-stimulating hormone, luteinizing hormone, and prolactin levels were all decreased below the reference range.

A definitive diagnosis of pituitary abscess syndrome occurs at necropsy. Typical necropsy findings include identification of a 3- to 5-cm encapsulated abscess in the area of the pituitary gland resulting in compression of adjacent cranial nerves **(Fig. 5)**.[169,176] Histologic findings are consistent with pyogranulomatous inflammation and necrosis.[72,169,177]

Treatment

Pituitary abscess syndrome is consistently fatal. Therefore, treatment is unrewarding and typically not recommended. A few reports[176,178] describe successful treatment with a combination of penicillin and streptomycin. However, these reports should be interpreted cautiously because the diagnosis of pituitary abscess was made presumptively based on clinical and neurologic signs and necropsy confirmation of pituitary abscess syndrome in similarly affected calves from the same groups. Details of treatment duration were not provided, but one author did report persistent neurologic abnormalities including moderate neck extension and paralysis.[176]

Prevention

Although there are no specific preventive measures for pituitary abscess syndrome, use of aseptic technique when inserting nose rings and prompt recognition and treatment of bacterial infections in other body systems may help to reduce the risk of pituitary abscess development. Producers should be aware of the potential risk of pituitary abscess associated with the use of nasal weaning flaps.

Summary

Pituitary abscess syndrome is an uncommon disease of ruminants that is thought to occur as a result of hematogenous spread of bacteria in the complex network of vessels known as the rete mirabile that surrounds the pituitary gland. Pituitary abscess syndrome typically results in neurologic abnormalities consistent with both cerebral and brainstem dysfunction. Brainstem lesions and accompanying cranial nerve deficits are often asymmetrical. Currently, there is no definitive antemortem diagnosis for pituitary abscess syndrome although imaging via CT scan or MRI or measurement of pituitary hormone levels may prove useful in the future. Definitive diagnosis is made at necropsy. Treatment is not recommended because pituitary abscess syndrome is consistently fatal. Pituitary abscess syndrome is an important differential diagnosis for animals exhibiting signs that localize to the brainstem, particularly when those signs are asymmetrical.

REFERENCES

1. Fenlon DR. Listeria monocytogenes in the natural environment. In: Ryser ET, Marth EH, editors. Listeria, listeriosis, and food safety. 2nd edition. New York: Marcel Dekker; 1999. p. 21–37.
2. Low JC, Donachie W. A review of Listeria monocytogenes and listeriosis. Vet J 1997;153:9–29.
3. Guyot H. Case report: two cases of ocular form of listeriosis in cattle herds. Cattle Pract 2011;19(1):61–4.
4. Peters M, Amtsberg G, Beckmann GT. The diagnosis of listeric encephalitis in ruminants using cultural and immunohistological techniques. I. Comparison of different selective media and cultural techniques to isolate Listeria spp. from the brains of ruminants. Zentralbl Veterinarmed B 1992;39:410–20 [in German].
5. Peters M, Hewicker-Trautwein M, Amtsberg G. The diagnosis of listeric encephalitis in ruminants using cultural and immunohistological techniques. II. Communication: immunohistological investigations on formalin-fixed paraffin sections. Zentralbl Veterinarmed B 1992;39:473–84 [in German].
6. Kathariou S. Listeria monocytogenes virulence and pathogenicity, a food perspective. J Food Prot 2002;65(11):1811–29.
7. Dhama K, Karthik K, Tiwari R, et al. Listeriosis in animals, its public health significance (food-borne zoonosis) and advances in diagnosis and control: a comprehensive review. Vet Q 2015;35(4):211–35.
8. Giannati-Stefanou A, Tsakos P, Bourtzi-Hatzopoulou E, et al. Study of microbiological aspects of meningoencephalitis due to Listeria spp. in ruminants. J Hellenic Vet Med Soc 2006;57(4):275–88.
9. Wardrope DD, Macleod NSM. Outbreak of listeria meningoencephalitis in young lambs. Vet Rec 1983;113:213–4.
10. Low JC, Wright F, McLaughlin J, et al. Serotyping and distribution of Listeria isolates from cases of ovine listeriosis. Vet Rec 1993;133:165–6.
11. Erdogan HM. Listerial keratoconjunctivitis and uveitis (silage eye). Vet Clin North Am Food Anim Pract 2010;26:505–10.
12. Garcia JA, Micheloud JF, Campero CM, et al. Enteric listeriosis in grazing steers supplemented with spoiled silage. J Vet Diagn Invest 2016;28(1):65–9.
13. Wesley IV, Larson DJ, Harmon KM, et al. A case report of sporadic ovine listerial meningoencephalitis in Iowa with an overview of livestock and human cases. J Vet Diagn Invest 2002;14:314–21.
14. Wilesmith JW. Epidemiology of ovine listeriosis in Great Britain. Vet Rec 1986; 119(19):467–70.
15. Morin DE. Brainstem and cranial nerve abnormalities: listeriosis, otitis media/interna, and pituitary abscess syndrome. Vet Clin North Am Food Anim Pract 2004;20:243–73.

16. Nash ML, Hungerford LL, Nash TG, et al. Epidemiology and economics of clinical listeriosis in a sheep flock. Prev Vet Med 1995;24:147–56.
17. Johnson GC, Maddox CW, Fales WH, et al. Epidemiologic evaluation of encephalitic listeriosis in goats. J Am Vet Med Assoc 1996;208:1695–9.
18. Barlow RM, McGorum B. Ovine listerial encephalitis: analysis, hypothesis and synthesis. Vet Rec 1985;116:233–6.
19. Green LE, Morgan KL. Descriptive epidemiology of listerial meningoencephalitis in housed lambs. Prev Vet Med 1994;18:79–87.
20. Rebhun WC, deLahunta A. Diagnosis and treatment of bovine listeriosis. J Am Vet Med Assoc 1982;180:395–8.
21. Rebuhn WC, Edwards RB. Challenging cases in internal medicine: what's your diagnosis? Vet Med 1992;87(7):640–4.
22. Schweizer G, Ehrensperger F, Torgerson P, et al. Clinical findings and treatment of 94 cattle presumptively diagnosed with listeriosis. Vet Rec 2016;158:588–92.
23. Molsan PG, Andrews GA, DeBey BM, et al. Listeriosis associated with silage feeding in six midwestern [USA] cattle herds. Large Anim Pract 1998;19(5):40–6.
24. Van Metre DC, Barrington GM, Parish SM, et al. Otitis media/interna and suppurative meningoencephalomyelitis associated with *Listeria monocytogenes* infection in a llama. J Am Vet Med Assoc 1991;199(2):236–40.
25. Butt MT, Weldon A, Step DL, et al. Encephalitic listeriosis in two adult llamas (*Lama glama*): clinical presentations, lesions, and immunofluorescence of *Listeria monocytogenes* in brainstem lesions. Cornell Vet 1991;81(3):251–8.
26. West HJ, Obwolo M. Bilateral facial paralysis in a cow with listeriosis. Vet Rec 1987;120:204–5.
27. Woo-Sam NH. Listeriosis in a Holstein cow. Can Vet J 1999;40:506–8.
28. Wiedmann M, Czajka J, Bsat N, et al. Diagnosis and epidemiological association of *Listeria monocytogenes* strains in two outbreaks of listerial encephalitis in small ruminants. J Clin Microbiol 1994;32(4):991–6.
29. Wiedmann M, Arvik T, Bruce JL, et al. Investigation of a listeriosis epizootic in sheep in New York state. Am J Vet Res 1997;58(7):733–7.
30. Vandegraaff R, Borland NA, Browning JW. An outbreak of Listerial meningoencephalitis in sheep. Aust Vet J 1981;57:94–6.
31. Blenden DC, Kampelmacher EH, Torres-Anjel MJ. Listeriosis. J Am Vet Med Assoc 1987;191(12):1546–51.
32. Vasquez-Boland JA, Dominguez L, Blanco M, et al. Epidemiologic investigation of a silage-associated epizootic of ovine listeric encephalitis, using a new Listeria-selective enumeration medium and phage typing. Am J Vet Res 1992;53(3):368–71.
33. Gates GA, Blenden DC, Kintner LD. Listeric myelitis in sheep. J Am Vet Med Assoc 1967;150(2):200–4.
34. Erdogan HM, Cetinkaya B, Green LE, et al. Prevalence, incidence, signs and treatment of clinical listeriosis in dairy cattle in England. Vet Rec 2001;149:289–93.
35. Braun U, Stehle C, Ehrensperger F. Clinical findings and treatment of listeriosis in 67 sheep and goats. Vet Rec 2002;150(1):38–42.
36. Scott PR. A field study of ovine listerial meningo-encephalitis with particular reference to cerebrospinal fluid analysis as an aid to diagnosis and prognosis. Br Vet J 1993;149:165–70.

37. Nightingale KK, Fortes ED, Ho AJ, et al. Evaluation of farm management practices as risk factors for clinical listeriosis and fecal shedding of *Listeria monocytogenes* in ruminants. J Am Vet Med Assoc 2005;227:1808–14.

38. Mohammed HO, Stipetic K, McDonough PL, et al. Identification of potential on-farm sources of *Listeria monocytogenes* in herds of dairy cattle. Am J Vet Res 2009;70:383–8.

39. Husu JR. Epidemiologic studies on the occurrence of *Listeria monocytogenes* in the feces of dairy cattle. J Vet Med B 1990;37:276–82.

40. Seaman JT, Carrigan MJ, Cockram FA, et al. An outbreak of listerial myelitis in sheep. Aust Vet J 1990;67:142–3.

41. Francoz D. Cranial nerve abnormalities. In: Anderson DE, Rings M, editors. Current veterinary therapy: food animal practice 5. St Louis (MO): Saunders Elsevier; 2009. p. 299–306.

42. Bundrant BN, Hutchins T, den Bakker HC, et al. Listeriosis outbreak in dairy cattle caused by an unusual *Listeria monocytogenesis* serotype 4b strain. J Vet Diagn Invest 2011;23:155–8.

43. Gronstol H. Listeriosis in sheep. Isolation of *Listeria monocytogenes* from grass silage. Acta Vet Scand 1979;20:492–7.

44. Irvin AD. The effect of pH on the multiplication of *Listeria monocytogenes* in grass silage media. Vet Rec 1968;82(4):115–6.

45. Killinger AH, Mansfield ME. Epizootiology of listeric infection in sheep. J Am Vet Med Assoc 1970;157(10):1318–24.

46. Ayars WH, Monke DR, Love B. An outbreak of encephalitic listeriosis in Holstein bulls. Bov Pract 1999;33(2):138–41.

47. Sargisson N. Health hazards associated with the feeding of big bale silage. In Practice 1993;15(6):291–7.

48. Duniere L, Sindou J, Chaucheyras-Durand F, et al. Silage processing and strategies to prevent persistence of undesirable microorganisms. Anim Feed Sci Technol 2013;182:1–15.

49. Fenlon DR. Rapid quantitative assessment of the distribution of listeria in silage implicated in a suspected outbreak of listeriosis in calves. Vet Rec 1986;118:240–2.

50. Brugère-Picoux J. Ovine listeriosis. Small Rum Res 2008;76(1/2):12–20.

51. Wood JS. Encephalitic listeriosis in a herd of goats. Can Vet J 1972;13(3):80–2.

52. Dijkstra RG. Listeria-encefalitis in cows through litter from a broiler-farm. Zentralbl Bakteriol Orig B 1976;161(4):383–5.

53. Ueno H, Yokota K, Arai T, et al. The prevalence of *Listeria monocytogenes* in the environment of dairy farms. Microbiol Immunol 1996;40(2):121–4.

54. Asahi O, Hosoda T, Akiyama Y. Studies on the mechanism of infection of the brain with *Listeria monocytogenes*. Am J Vet Res 1957;18:147–57.

55. Asahi O. Pathogenesis of encephalitic listeriosis: invasion of nerve fibers by Listeria monocytogenes. In: Gray ML, editor. Proceedings of the 2nd symposium on listeric infection. Bozeman (MT): Aircraft Printers; 1963. p. 100–8.

56. George LW. Listeriosis (circling disease; silage disease; Listeria monocytogenes infection). In: Smith BP, editor. Large animal internal medicine. 5th edition. St Louis (MO): Saunders Elsevier; 2015. p. 969–71.

57. Charlton KM. Spontaneous listeric encephalitis in sheep. Electron microscopic studies. Vet Pathol 1977;14:429–34.

58. Charlton KM, Garcia MM. Spontaneous listeric encephalitis and neuritis in sheep. Light microscopic studies. Vet Pathol 1977;14:297–313.

59. Osebold JW. Some aspects of the pathogenesis of listeriosis. In: Gray ML, editor. Proceedings of the 2nd symposium on listeric infection. Bozeman (MT): Aircraft Printers; 1963. p. 109–13.

60. Akiyama Y, Asahi O, Hosoda T. Experimental infection of rats, guinea pigs, hamsters, dogs, and cats with Listeria monocytogenes through a branch of nervus trigeminus. Nat Health Inst Q 1961;1:20–31.

61. Otter A, Blakemore WF. Observation on the presence of Listeria monocytogenes in axons. Acta Microbiol Hung 1989;36(2–3):125–31.

62. Henke D, Rupp S, Gaschen V, et al. Listeria monocytogenes spreads within the brain by actin-based intra-axonal migration. Infect Immun 2015;83:2409–19.

63. Anthal E-A, Marit Loberg E, Bracht P, et al. Evidence of intraaxonal spread of Listeria monocytogenes from the periphery to the central nervous system. Brain Pathol 2001;11:432–8.

64. Orndorff PE, Hamrick TS, Washington Smoak I, et al. Host and bacterial factors in listeriosis pathogenesis. Vet Microbiol 2006;114:1–15.

65. Southwick FS, Purich DL. Intracellular pathogenesis of listeriosis. N Engl J Med 1996;334(12):770–6.

66. Evans K, Smith M, McDonough P, et al. Eye infections due to Listeria monocytogenes in three cows and one horse. J Vet Diagn Invest 2004;16:464–9.

67. Scott PR. Clinical diagnosis of ovine listeriosis. Small Rum Res 2013;110(2-3):138–41.

68. Roeder BL, Johnson JW, Cash WC. Paradoxic vestibular syndrome in a cow with a metastatic brain tumour. Compend Contin Educ Pract Vet 1990;12(8):1175–81.

69. Schweizer G, Fuhrer B, Braun U. Signs of spinal cord disease in two heifers caused by Listeria monocytogenes. Vet Rec 2004;154:54–5.

70. Pfister H, Remer KA, Brcic M, et al. Inducible nitric oxide synthase and nitrotyrosine in listeric encephalitis: a cross-species study in ruminants. Vet Pathol 2002;39:190–9.

71. Wiedmann M. Listeria monocytogenes: transmission and disease in ruminants. Proceedings of the 26th American College of Veterinary Internal Medicine. San Antonio (TX), June 4–7, 2008. p. 255–7.

72. Perdrizet JA, Dinsmore P. Pituitary abscess syndrome. Compend Contin Educ Pract Vet 1986;8(6):S311–9.

73. Roels S, Dobly A, De Sloovere J, et al. Listeria monocytogenes-associated meningo-encephalitis in cattle clinically suspected of bovine spongiform encephalopathy in Belgium (1998-2006). Vlaams Diergeneeskundig Tijdschrift 2009;78(3):177–81.

74. Scott PR, Henshaw CJ, Clarke CJ. Flaccid oesophageal paralysis in a Friesian heifer associated with encephalitis. Vet Rec 1994;135:482–3.

75. Ferrouillet C, Fecteau G, Higgins R, et al. Analyse du liquide cephalo-rachidien pour le diagnostic des atteintes du systeme nerveux des bovins (Analysis of cerebrospinal fluid for diagnosis of nervous system diseases in cattle). Point Veterinaire 1998;29(194):783–8.

76. Scarratt WK. Ovine listeric encephalitis. Comp Cont Edu Pract Vet 1987;9(1):F28–33.

77. Stokol T, Divers TJ, Arrigan JW, et al. Cerebrospinal fluid findings in cattle with central nervous system disorders: a retrospective study of 102 cases (1990-2008). Vet Clin Pathol 2009;38(1):103–12.

78. El-Boshy ME, El-Khodery SA, Gadalla HA, et al. Prognostic significance of selected immunological and biochemical parameters in the cerebrospinal fluid of Ossimi sheep with encephalitic listeriosis. Small Rum Res 2012;104:179–84.

79. Peters M, Pohlenz J, Jaton K, et al. Studies of the detection of *Listeria monocytogenes* by culture and PCR in cerebrospinal fluid samples from ruminants with listeric encephalitis. J Vet Med B 1995;42:84–8.

80. Oevermann A, Di Palma S, Doherr MG, et al. Neuropathogenesis of naturally occurring encephalitis caused by *Listeria monocytogenes* in ruminants. Brain Pathol 2010;20:378–90.

81. Allen AL, Goupil BA, Valentine BA. A retrospective study of brain lesions in goats submitted to three veterinary diagnostic laboratories. J Vet Diagn Invest 2013; 25(4):482–9.

82. Johnson GC, Fales WH, Maddox CW, et al. Evaluation of laboratory tests for confirming the diagnosis of encephalitic listeriosis in ruminants. J Vet Diagn Invest 1995;7:223–8.

83. Weinstock D, Horton SB, Rowland PH. Rapid diagnosis of *Listeria monocytogenes* by immunohistochemistry in formalin-fixed brain tissue. Vet Pathol 1995;32:193–5.

84. Campero CM, Odeon AC, Cipolla AL, et al. Demonstration of *Listeria monocytogenes* by immunohistochemistry in formalin-fixed brain tissues from natural cases of ovine and bovine encephalitis. J Vet Med B 2002;49:379–83.

85. Loeb E. Encephalitic listeriosis in ruminants: immunohistochemistry as a diagnostic tool. J Vet Med A Physiol Pathol Clin Med 2004;51:453–5.

86. Marco A, Ramos JA, Dominguez L, et al. Immunocytochemical detection of *Listeria monocytogenes* in tissue with the peroxidase-antiperoxidase technique. Vet Pathol 1988;25:385–7.

87. Baetz AL, Wesley IV. Detection of anti-listeriolysin O in dairy cattle experimentally infected with *Listeria monocytogenes*. J Vet Diagn Invest 1995;7:82–6.

88. Low JC, Donachie W. Clinical and serum antibody responses of lambs to infection by *Listeria monocytogenes*. Res Vet Sci 1991;51:185–92.

89. Miettinen A, Husu J, Tuomi J. Serum antibody response to *Listeria monocytogenes*, listerial excretion, and clinical characteristics in experimentally infected goats. J Clin Microbiol 1990;28(2):340–3.

90. Boerlin P, Boerlin-Petzold F, Jemmi T. Use of listeriolysin O and internalin A in a seroepidemiological study of listeriosis in Swiss dairy cows. J Clin Microbiol 2003;41(3):1055–61.

91. Aittoniemi J, Husu J, Jaakkolat O, et al. Clinical determinants and time course of serum antibody response against listeriolysin O in experimental listeriosis. Serodiagn Immunother Infect Dis 1995;7(3):105–8.

92. Amagliani G, Giammarini C, Omiccioli E, et al. A combination of diagnostic tools for rapid screening of ovine listeriosis. Res Vet Sci 2006;81:185–9.

93. Dreyer M, Thomann A, Bottcher S, et al. Outbreak investigation identifies a single *Listeria monocytogenes* strain in sheep with different clinical manifestation, soil and water. Vet Microbiol 2015;179:69–75.

94. Wiedmann M, Bruce JL, Knorr R, et al. Ribotype diversity of *Listeria monocytogenes* strains associated with outbreaks of listeriosis in ruminants. J Clin Microbiol 1996;34(5):1086–90.

95. Arimi SM, Ryser ET, Pritchard TJ, et al. Diversity of Listeria ribotypes recovered from dairy cattle, silage, and dairy processing environments. J Food Prot 1997; 60(7):811–6.

96. Low JC, Chalmers RM, Donachie W, et al. Pyrolysis mass spectrometry of *Listeria monocytogenes* isolates from sheep. Res Vet Sci 1992;53:64–7.

97. Hof H. Therapeutic activities of antibiotics in listeriosis. Infection 1991;19(Suppl 4):S229–33.

98. Hof H. An update on the medical management of listeriosis. Expert Opin Pharmacother 2004;5(8):1727–35.

99. Srinivasan V, Nam HM, Nguyen LT, et al. Prevalence of antimicrobial resistance genes in *Listeria monocytogenes* isolated from dairy farms. Foodborne Pathog Dis 2005;2(3):201–11.

100. Charpentier E, Gerbaud G, Jacquet C, et al. Incidence of antibiotic resistance in *Listeria* species. J Infect Dis 1995;172:277–81.

101. Rebhun WC. Listeriosis. Vet Clin North Am Food Anim Pract 1987;3(1):75–83.

102. Wesley IV, Bryner JH, Van Der Maaten MJ, et al. Effects of dexamethasone on shedding of *Listeria monocytogenes* in dairy cattle. Am J Vet Res 1989; 50(12):2009–13.

103. Garner D, Kathariou S. Fresh produce-associated listeriosis outbreaks, sources of concern, teachable moments, and insights. J Food Prot 2016;79(2):337–44.

104. Farber JM, Peterkin PI. Listeria monocytogenes, a food-borne pathogen. Microbiol Rev 1991;55(3):476–511.

105. Ryser ET. Foodborne listeriosis. In: Ryser ET, Marth EH, editors. Listeria, listeriosis, and food safety. 2nd edition. New York: Marcel Dekker; 1999. p. 299–358.

106. Ladds PW, Dennis SM, Njoku CO, et al. Pathology of listeric infection in domestic animals. Vet Bull 1974;44(2):67–73.

107. Gudding R, Gronstol H, Larsen HJ. Vaccination against listeriosis in sheep. Vet Rec 1985;117:89–90.

108. Linde K, Fthenakis GC, Lippmann R, et al. The efficacy of a live *Listeria monocytogenes* combined serotype 1/2a and serotype 4b vaccine. Vaccine 1995; 13(10):923–6.

109. Szemeredi GA. Ten year's experience with inactivated vaccine against listeriosis of sheep. Acta Microbiologica Hungarica 1989;36(2–3):327–30.

110. De Lahunta A, Glass E. Vestibular system: special proprioception. In: De Lahunta A, Glass E, editors. Veterinary neuroanatomy and clinical neurology. 3rd edition. St Louis (MO): Saunders Elsevier; 2009. p. 147–8, 319-29.

111. Nation PN, Frelier PF, Gifford GA, et al. Otitis in feedlot cattle. Can Vet J 1983;24: 238.

112. McEwen SA, Hulland TJ. *Haemophilus somnus*-induced otitis and meningitis in a heifer. Can Vet J 1985;26:7–8.

113. Yeruham I, Elad D, Liberboim M. Clinical and microbiological study of an otitis media outbreak in calves in a dairy herd. J Vet Med B 1999;46:145–50.

114. Vestweber JG. Otitis media/interna in cattle. Compend Contin Educ Pract Vet 1999;21(1):S34–7.

115. Francoz D, Fecteau G, Desrochers A, et al. Otitis media in dairy calves: a retrospective study of 15 cases (1987-2002). Can Vet J 2004;45:661–6.

116. Bernier Gosselin V, Francoz D, Babkine M, et al. A retrospective study of 29 cases of otitis media/interna in dairy calves. Can Vet J 2012;53:957–62.

117. Walz PH, Mullaney TP, Render JA, et al. Otitis media in preweaned Holstein dairy calves in Michigan due to *Mycoplasma bovis*. J Vet Diagn Invest 1997; 9:250–4.

118. Lamm CG, Munson L, Thurmond MC, et al. *Mycoplasma* otitis in California calves. J Vet Diagn Invest 2004;16:397–402.

119. Foster AP, Naylor RD, Howie NM, et al. Mycoplasma bovis and otitis in dairy calves in the United Kingdom. Vet J 2009;179:455–7.
120. Jensen R, Maki LR, Lauerman LH, et al. Cause and pathogenesis of middle ear infection in young feedlot cattle. J Am Vet Med Assoc 1983;182(9):967–72.
121. Duarte ER, Hamdan JS. Otitis in cattle: an aetiological review. J Vet Med B 2004; 51:1–7.
122. Bertone L, Bellino C, Alborali GL, et al. Clinical-pathological findings of otitis media and media-interna in calves and (clinical) evaluation of a standardized therapeutic protocol. BMC Vet Res 2015;11:297.
123. DaMassa AJ. Prevalence of Mycoplasmas and mites in the external auditory meatus of goats. Calif Vet 1983;37(12):10–7.
124. Cottew GS, Yeats FR. Mycoplasmas and mites in the ears of clinically normal goats. Aust Vet J 1982;59:77–81.
125. Leask R, Blignaut DJC, Grobler MJ. *Corynebacterium pseudotuberculosis* associated with otitis media-interna in goats. J S Afr Vet Assoc 2013;84(1):969.
126. Jensen R, Pierson RE, Weibel JL, et al. Middle ear infection in feedlot lambs. J Am Vet Med Assoc 1982;181(8):805–7.
127. Davies IH, Done SH. Necrotic dermatitis and otitis media associated with Pseudomonas aeruginosa in sheep following dipping. Vet Rec 1993;132(18):460–1.
128. Henderson JP, McCullough WP. Otitis media in suckler calves. Vet Rec 1993; 132(1):24.
129. Msolla P. Bovine parasitic otitis: an up-to-date review. Vet Annual 1989;29:73–7.
130. Otero Negrete J, Jaramillo Meza L, Miranda Morales RE, et al. Association *of Raillietia caprae* with the presence of *Mycoplasmas* in the external ear canal of goats. Prev Vet Med 2009;92:150–3.
131. Msolla P, Semuguruka WD, Kasuku AA, et al. Clinical observations of bovine parasitic otitis in Tanzania. Trop Anim Health Prod 1993;25:15–8.
132. Duarte ER, Melo MM, Hamdan JS. Epidemiological aspects of bovine parasitic otitis caused by *Rhabditis* spp. and/or *Raillietia* spp. in the state of Minas Gerais, Brazil. Vet Parasitol 2001;101:45–52.
133. Ladds PW, Copeman DB, Daniels P, et al. *Raillietia auris* and otitis media in cattle in northern Queensland. Aust Vet J 1972;48:532–3.
134. Wilson J, Brewer BD. Vestibular disease in a goat. Compend Contin Educ Pract Vet 1984;6(3):S179–82.
135. Heffner RS, Heffner HE. Occurrence of the cattle ear mite (*Raillietia auris*) in southeastern Kansas. Cornell Vet 1983;73(2):193–9.
136. DaMassa AJ. The ear canal as a culture site for demonstration of mycoplasmas in clinically normal goats. Aust Vet J 1990;67(6):267–9.
137. Madsen LW, Svensmark B, Elvestad K, et al. Otitis interna is a frequent sequela to *Streptococcus suis* meningitis in pigs. Vet Pathol 2001;38:190–5.
138. Mayhew J. Infectious, inflammatory, and immune diseases (otitis media and otitis interna). In: Mayhew J, editor. Large animal neurology. 2nd edition. Chichester (United Kingdom): Wiley-Blackwell; 2009. p. 235–7.
139. Shimada A, Adachi T, Umemura T, et al. A pathologic and bacteriologic study on otitis media in swine. Vet Pathol 1992;29(4):337–42.
140. Friis NF, Kokotovic B, Svensmark B. *Mycoplasma hyorhinis* isolation from cases of otitis media in piglets. Acta Vet Scand 2002;43:191–3.
141. Van Biervliet J, Perkins GA, Woodie B, et al. Clinical signs, computed tomographic imaging, and management of chronic otitis media/interna in dairy calves. J Vet Intern Med 2004;18:907–10.

142. Yeruham I, Elad D. Acute bilateral suppurative otitis media in a dairy cow. Can Vet J 2004;45:779.
143. Rademacher G, Schels H, Dirksen G. Enzootic otitis in a group of calves. Tierarztl Prax 1991;19:253–7.
144. Koenig JB, Watrous BJ, Kaneps AJ, et al. Otitis media in a llama. J Am Vet Med Assoc 2001;218(10):1619–23.
145. Galvan N, Middleton JR, Cook C, et al. Otitis interna, media, and externa with destruction of the left tympanic bulla and subluxation and septic arthritis of the left temporomandibular joint in an alpaca (Vicugna pacos). Can Vet J 2013;54:283–5.
146. Macleod NSM, Wiener G, Barlow RM, et al. Factors involved in middle ear infection (otitis media) in lambs. Vet Rec 1972;91(15):360–1.
147. Maunsell F, Brown MB, Powe J, et al. Oral inoculation of young dairy calves with Mycoplasma bovis results in colonization of tonsils, development of otitis media and local immunity. PLoS One 2012;7(9):e44523.
148. Baba AI, Rotaru O, Rapuntean G. Middle ear infection in suckling and weaned calves. Morphol Embryol 1988;34(4):271–5.
149. Maeda T, Shibahara T, Kimura K, et al. Mycoplasma bovis-associated suppurative otitis media and pneumonia in bull calves. J Comp Pathol 2003;129:100–10.
150. Maunsell F, Donavan GA. Mycoplasma bovis infections in young calves. Vet Clin Food Anim Pract 2009;25:139–77.
151. Finnen A, Blond L, Francoz D, et al. Comparison of computed tomography and routine radiography of the tympanic bullae in the diagnosis of otitis media in the calf. J Vet Intern Med 2011;25:143–7.
152. Bernier Gosselin V, Babkine M, Gains MJ, et al. Validation of an ultrasound imaging technique of the tympanic bullae for the diagnosis of otitis media in calves. J Vet Intern Med 2014;28:1594–601.
153. Leite PVB, Leite LB, Cunha AP da, et al. Clinical aspects and dynamics of auricular parasitosis in Gir cattle. Pres Vet Bras 2013;33(3):319–25.
154. Hazell SL, Greenwood PE, Adams BS. Isolation of mycoplasmas from the external ear canal of a cow. Aust Vet J 1986;63(4):129–30.
155. Sumner JP, Mueller T, Clapp KS, et al. Modified ear canal ablation and lateral bulla osteotomy for management of otitis media in an alpaca. Vet Surg 2012;41:273–7.
156. Ferrell ST, Valverde C, Phillips LG Jr. Chronic otitis externa/media with total ear canal ablation and bulla curettage in a north American bison (bison bison). J Zoo Wildl Med 2001;32(3):393–5.
157. Bernier Gosselin V, Babkine M, Francoz D. Ultrasonography of the tympanic bullae and larynx in cattle. Vet Clin Food Anim Pract 2016;32:119–31.
158. Nunes VA. Post-mortem technique for examination of auditive system applied to study of bovine otitis. Arq Esc Vet UFMG 1975;27(2):155–61.
159. Ayling R, Nicolas R, Hogg R, et al. Mycoplasma bovis isolated from brain tissue of calves. Vet Rec 2005;156:391–2.
160. Msolla P, Falmer-Hansen J, Musemakweli J, et al. Treatment of bovine parasitic otitis using ivermectin. Trop Anim Health Prod 1985;17:166–8.
161. Francoz D, Fortin M, Fecteau G, et al. Determination of Mycoplasma bovis susceptibilities against six antimicrobial agents using the E test method. Vet Microbiol 2005;105:57–64.
162. Rosenbusch RF, Kinyon JM, Apley M, et al. In vitro antimicrobial inhibition profiles of Mycoplasma bovis isolates from various regions of the United States from 2002 to 2003. J Vet Diagn Invest 2005;17:436–41.

163. Apley MD, Fajt VR. Feedlot therapeutics. Vet Clin North Am Food Anim Pract 1998;14(2):291–313.

164. Poetker DM, Ubell ML, Kerschner JE. Disease severity in patients referred to pediatric otolaryngologists with a diagnosis of otitis media. Int J Pediatr Otorhinolaryngol 2006;70:311–7.

165. Schnepper R. Practice tips. In: Proceedings of the 35th Annual Conference of the American Association of Bovine Practitioners. Madison (WI), September 26–28, 2002. p. 26–8.

166. Villarroel A, Heller MC, Lane VM, et al. Imaging study of myringotomy in dairy calves. Bov Pract 2006;40(1):14–7.

167. Pardon B, Hostens M, Ducahteau L, et al. Impact of respiratory disease, diarrhea, otitis and arthritis on mortality and carcass traits in white veal calves. BMC Vet Res 2013;9:79.

168. Butler JA, Sickles SA, Johanns CJ, et al. Pasteurization of discard Mycoplasma mastitis milk used to feed calves: thermal effects on various Mycoplasma. J Dairy Sci 2000;83:2285–8.

169. Loretti AP, Ilha MRS, Riet-Correa G, et al. Pituitary abscess syndrome in calves following injury of the nasal septum by a plastic device used to prevent suckling. Pesqui Vet Bras 2003;23(1):39–46.

170. Müller KR, Blutke A, Matiasek K, et al. Pituitary abscess syndrome in a Simmental heifer. Vet Rec Case Rep 2014;2(1):e000041.

171. Yeruham I, Orgad U, Avidar Y, et al. Pituitary abscess and high urea concentration as causes of neurological signs in a cow. Rev Med Vet 2002;153(12): 829–31.

172. Lomas ST, Hazell SL. The isolation of *Mycoplasma arginini* from a pituitary abscess in a goat. Aust Vet J 1983;60(9):281–2.

173. Dabak M, Eroksuz Y, Baydar E, et al. Decreased pituitary hormone levels in a sheep with pituitary abscess. J Appl Anim Res 2016;44(1):5–8.

174. Reilly L, Habecker P, Beech J, et al. Pituitary abscess and basilar empyema in 4 horses. Equine Vet J 1994;26(5):424–6.

175. Su Y-H, Chen Y, Tseng S-H. Pituitary abscess. J Clin Neurosci 2006;13(10): 1038–41.

176. Fernandes CG, Schild AL, Riet-Correa F, et al. Pituitary abscess in young calves associated with the use of a controlled suckling device. J Vet Diagn Invest 2000; 12(1):70–1.

177. Rech RR, Rissi RR, Silva MC, et al. Histomorphology of the Gasserian ganglion, carotid rete mirabile and pituitary gland in cattle: a study of 199 cases. Pesquisa Veterinaria Brasileira 2006;26(2):105–11.

178. Camara ACL, Borges JRJ, Godoy RF, et al. Pituitary abscess syndrome in calves from Mid-Western. Pesquisa Veterinaria Brasileira 2009;29(11):925–30.

179. Moriwaki M, Watase H, Fukumoto M, et al. Exophthalmos due to rete mirabile abscess caused by infection with *Corynebacterium pyogenes* in cattle. Natl Inst Anim Health Q 1973;13(1):14–22.

180. El-Khodery S, Yamada K, Aoki D, et al. Brain abscess in a Japanese black calf: utility of computed tomography (CT). J Vet Med Sci 2008;70(7):727–30.

Spinal Cord and Peripheral Nerve Abnormalities of the Ruminant

Amanda K. Hartnack, DVM, MS, BA

KEYWORDS

- Peripheral nerve injury • Spinal cord injury • Spinal cord trauma • Paresis • Paralysis
- Parasitic

KEY POINTS

- Disorders of the spinal cord in ruminants are most often associated with infectious or traumatic causes, including vertebral body abscess or vertebral fracture, and are commonly associated with a grave prognosis.
- Parasitic migration may result in spinal cord damage and is most often associated with *Hypoderma bovis* and *Parelaphostrongylus tenuis*.
- Peripheral nerve abnormalities are commonly traumatic in nature, with the radial nerve being commonly damaged in the forelimb and the sciatic or obturator commonly associated with calving injury in the hind limb.

Disorders of the spinal cord and peripheral nerves in ruminants are most commonly associated with infectious or traumatic causes, with clinical signs varying depending on the severity and location of the lesion.

Differential diagnoses for animals with signs of spinal cord damage include vertebral body abscess or osteomyelitis, spinal abscess, spinal trauma, parasitic migration, neoplasia, or congenital vertebral or spinal cord abnormality.

SPINAL CORD: INFECTIOUS

Vertebral body infection and epidural spinal abscesses occur regularly in ruminants, occurring in both young and adult animals. These conditions are seen more commonly in animals less than 12 months of age than in adult animals. Vertebral body osteomyelitis generally occurs following hematogenous spread of bacteria from infectious processes distant from the vertebral bodies. These disease processes may include

Disclosure Statement: The author has nothing to disclose.
Food Animal Surgery, Department of Large Animal Clinical Sciences, Texas A&M University, 4475 TAMU, College Station, TX 77843, USA
E-mail address: ahartnack@cvm.tamu.edu

pulmonary or umbilical infections in calves, bacteremia secondary to septicemia in calves, or localized abscesses.[1,2] In lambs, abscesses or cauda equina syndrome secondary to ascending infection may be associated with tail docking.

Clinical signs may appear acutely as in the case of a pathologic fracture or insidiously with extension of osteomyelitis. Abscesses may be located in the vertebral body, intervertebral disk space, or paravertebral. Because of the association with other diseases, such as pneumonia, affected animals may have a history of disease or ill thrift.

Diagnosis is based on a combination of history and clinical signs, with radiographic imaging often providing a definitive diagnosis. Clinical signs, of course, depend on the site of the compressive lesion. In about 50% of cases, more than one vertebral body is affected; lesions seem to be distributed between cervical, thoracic, and lumbar regions.[3] Other imaging techniques that may be helpful in the diagnosis include computed tomography (CT), MRI, and myelography.

Abnormalities on a complete blood count or serum chemistry may include elevations in fibrinogen, globulin, and white blood cell counts, all consistent with a chronic infection. Although a cerebrospinal fluid (CSF) tap may be helpful in ruling out other diseases, findings are often nonspecific. CSF may be normal or may reveal a pleocytosis (mononuclear or neutrophilic).[4] Uncommonly, the abscess is penetrated while performing a CSF tap, resulting in aspiration of purulent material.

Necropsy examination may reveal gross signs of spinal cord compression, and histologic examination of the spinal cord reveals pressure necrosis and Wallerian degeneration as well as localized meningitis.[3]

Because of the poor prognosis, treatment is rarely attempted. However, laminectomy has been reported as a successful treatment of an epidural abscess in a calf.[5] In most situations, prevention of the condition is emphasized. Prevention strategies include ensuring adequate passive transfer in neonates and excellent hygiene to prevent other predisposing conditions, such as pneumonia or umbilical infection.

TRAUMA

In both young and adult ruminants, spinal cord trauma is most commonly associated with vertebral fractures, though the cause of these fractures is different between the two groups. Spinal cord trauma may also occur in the absence of a vertebral body fracture due to soft tissue swelling adjacent to the spinal cord or from direct injury to the cord.

Although vertebral fractures are rare, they generally involve the vertebral body and are often associated with severe neurologic signs. Signs, as with all spinal cord lesions, depend on the location and severity of injury. In adults, these fractures may be secondary to direct trauma, such as riding injuries and restraint for processing.[6–8] More commonly, however, vertebral fractures are seen in neonates and are generally associated with assisted delivery during dystocia.[9–11] Spinal cord compression may also occur secondary to fracture callus formation, resulting in a potentially insidious onset of signs. Pathologic fractures of the vertebrae in ruminants have been associated with osteomyelitis or nutritional imbalances, such as calcium, phosphorus, vitamin D, and copper.[12–16] In both calves and small ruminants, predator attacks may also be a cause of spinal cord trauma.

Diagnosis of vertebral fracture is based on clinical signs, history of trauma (if known), and radiographic confirmation. Rectal examination in adult cattle may reveal a step lesion if a vertebral fracture is present. If a nutritional cause is suspected, radiographic appearance of the skeleton, feed analysis, and supporting laboratory work can be used to confirm and definitively diagnose the cause. Spinal cord trauma without vertebral fracture is more difficult to diagnose, as advanced imaging techniques must be used. Myelography, CT, or MRI may aid in the definitive diagnosis of suspected lesions. Because of size constraints, CT or MRI is not possible in adult cattle and myelography is of limited use.

CSF analysis is variable in animals with spinal cord trauma. Changes may include histiocytic pleocytosis, elevated protein, erythrophagia, or xanthochromia. Depending on the site and severity of the lesion, CSF analysis following traumatic spinal cord injury may be normal.[4]

Treatment of these types of injuries is largely unsuccessful and is rarely attempted in food producing animals because of both cost and size considerations. Vertebral fractures require internal fixation, which is rarely attempted. Traditionally, use of corticosteroids has been a mainstay of treatment in animals without vertebral fracture; however, use of corticosteroids for acute spinal injury in humans is no longer recommended.[17]

NEOPLASIA

Lymphosarcoma is the most common neoplastic process affecting the bovine spinal cord, as the spinal column is one of the top predilection sites for clinical bovine lymphosarcoma.[18,19] Lymphosarcoma tumors tend to be extradural in nature, causing compression of the spinal cord. More than half of the cases reported in a recent study affected the lumbar, sacral, and cauda equina regions, leading to clinical signs of hind-end ataxia and/or weakness.[18] However, tumors can occur in any region of the spinal column, and clinical signs will vary depending on the location of the lesion and the severity of cord compression.

Diagnosis of spinal lymphosarcoma can be challenging. Physical examination and clinical history are key in the diagnosis; however, a definitive antemortem diagnosis of spinal lymphosarcoma is rare. Rectal examination may reveal enlarged sublumbar lymph nodes, which raises the index of suspicion. Although a negative bovine leukemia virus test may be useful in eliminating clinical lymphosarcoma as a differential, a positive test will not confirm the diagnosis. Likewise, a complete blood count with a lymphocytosis may raise the index of suspicion but is not diagnostic in and of itself. CSF analysis has been reported to have 19% sensitivity, making it a potentially valuable diagnostic in some cases.[18] CSF taps consistent with lymphosarcoma are thought to result from the needle passing directly through the tumor, as these tumors tend to be extradural.

As with many other spinal cord abnormalities in ruminants, prognosis is grave. Corticosteroids may result in temporary improvement of symptoms; however, euthanasia is recommended.

PARASITIC MIGRATION

There are a few parasitic causes of spinal cord injury in ruminant animals, most notably migration of *Hypoderma bovis* in cattle and *Parelaphostrongylus tenuis* (meningeal worm) in other ruminants, including cattle.[20–24] Cases of *Parelaphostrongylus tenuis* involving cattle are, however, extremely rare, with New World camelids appearing most sensitive to infection.[25]

Hypoderma bovis (heel fly) larvae migrate through the epidural fat in cattle, leading to inflammation and varying degrees of clinical signs, with the lumbosacral spinal cord preferentially affected. This condition is relatively rare because of the widespread use of avermectin parasiticides. CSF tap may reveal an eosinophilia; however, because of the extradural location of the parasite, CSF may also be normal. Definitive diagnosis is made on necropsy examination. If treatment is attempted, it is based on decreasing inflammation using nonsteroidal antiinflammatory drugs or corticosteroids.

Parelaphostrongylus tenuis (meningeal worm) results in neurologic deficits secondary to migration of the larvae in aberrant hosts, such as New World camelids and small ruminants. This disease is endemic to North America, particularly in locations with large populations of white-tailed deer, the natural definitive host of the parasite. The parasite is passed to livestock via a snail or slug, the intermediate host. Disease occurs most often in the fall; however, infection can occur year round, particularly in wet environments.[26,27]

Following infection with *Parelaphostrongylus tenuis*, the parasite enters the parenchyma of the spinal cord, causing an inflammatory response. Onset of disease generally occurs 4 to 8 weeks after infection.[25,28] The inflammatory response in the spinal cord leads to the clinical signs, which are most commonly reported as hind limb ataxia with posterior paresis.[27,29–31] Signs may be unilateral and often progress to paresis and recumbency leading to death or euthanasia; however, spontaneous recovery has been reported.[27–29] Migration of the larvae to the brain has also been reported, resulting in signs of cerebral damage.

Antemortem diagnosis is based on clinical signs and the results of CSF analysis, with eosinophilic pleiocytosis being a hallmark finding.[32] However, lymphocytic pleocytosis has been reported in chronic infections in cattle.[22]

Necropsy examination of animals that died or were euthanized can provide a definitive diagnosis. Histopathology of the spinal cord may reveal the parasite within the parenchyma, and often linear tracks of hemorrhage, axonal degeneration, linear glial scars, or axonal necrosis and swelling are noted. Lymphocytic and plasmacytic and/or eosinophilic infiltrates have also been reported.[23,25,29]

Treatment consists of anthelmintic administration along with administration of antiinflammatory drugs. Although there is much anecdotal evidence that these treatment regimens work, studies demonstrating efficacy of treatment is lacking. Ivermectin, fenbendazole, or moxidectin alone or in combination have been used, with levamisole being the only anthelmintic with no reported success.[33]

NUTRITIONAL/TOXIC

The most common nutritional deficiency resulting in spinal cord damage is copper. Copper deficiency in kids and lambs during the prenatal or immediate postnatal period results in a condition known as enzootic ataxia (swayback). Animals are generally affected between birth and 4 months of age. Copper deficiency results in loss of myelin in the spinal cord (Wallerian degeneration).[34,35] Lesions may also be present in the cerebrum and cerebellum.

Diagnosis is based on clinical signs and necropsy examination, with low liver copper levels supporting the diagnosis. Concentration of copper in the blood may give an idea of deficiency as low levels indicate depletion in the liver; however, these values may be unreliable. Treatment with copper is ineffective because of impaired fetal development, and prepartum dietary changes in the adult ewes are necessary to prevent further cases.

Another neurodegenerative disease affecting cattle, sheep, and goats is chronic exposure to certain organophosphates, which is known as a dying back axonopathy. Clinical signs generally begin days to weeks following exposure, preferentially affecting the hind limbs and progressing to recumbency.[36] No treatment exists for this condition.

CONGENITAL

Several congenital spinal cord anomalies have been reported, including spina bifida, spinal dysraphism, and segmental aplasia of the spinal cord.[37–39] These anomalies most often result in stillbirth or require euthanasia shortly after birth because of the severity of the clinical signs or presence of other abnormalities.

Spina bifida is the result of incomplete closure of the dorsal laminae of the vertebrae, which form the vertebral arch. Spina bifida occulta is a defect of one or more vertebral arches, without exposure of the meninges or spinal cord. Spina bifida aperta is a failure of closure of the neural tube, resulting in visible defects, such as meningocele. Spina bifida cystica features a visible defect with a CSF-filled cyst. Diagnosis is based on clinical signs and physical examination. Radiographs may be helpful in the diagnosis of spinal bifida occulta.

Spinal dysraphisms represent any malformation of the spinal cord and may vary in degree of severity and locations within a single spinal cord. Spinal dysraphisms and spina bifida have been reported in several cattle breeds, with many of the defects being associated with postural abnormalities, including kyphoscoliosis and arthrogryposis.[37]

Prognosis is grave for animals born alive and euthanasia is recommended.

PERIPHERAL NERVE ABNORMALITIES

Peripheral nerve abnormalities are most often associated with trauma or are the result of myopathy in recumbent cattle. In calves and small ruminants, injections and trauma from a predator attack may also cause peripheral nerve injury.

FORELIMB

Radial nerve paralysis is common in adult cattle, particularly secondary to prolonged recumbency or squeeze chute injuries.

RADIAL NERVE

The radial nerve arises from the C7-T1 nerve roots and innervates extensors of the elbow, carpus, and digits as well as a flexor of the shoulder. Damage to the radial nerve occurs commonly in adult cattle and is generally unilateral. Animals most often present unable to bear weight on or dragging the affected forelimb, with a dropped elbow and partially flexed carpus and fetlock. With distal damage to the radial nerve, the triceps muscle may still be functional, resulting in minimal elbow drop. With severe injury to the radial nerve, there may be analgesia of the dorsal surface of the foot. Although large cattle may be unable to rise, smaller cattle and small ruminants may rise but place no weight on the limb.

Common causes of radial nerve paralysis include prolonged recumbency leading to a myopathy-compartmentalization syndrome, getting a forelimb trapped in a fence or feeder, excessive force placed on the distal neck and shoulder in a head catch, or falling on a hard, slick surface. Differential diagnoses include humeral fracture, olecranon fracture, and septic arthritis of the elbow joint.

Following damage to the radial nerve, the limb can be bandaged or splinted to maintain extension of the carpus and fetlock, allowing the animal to bear weight on the limb. This treatment will also help prevent abrasions to the dorsal surface of the fetlock. Additional treatment includes administration of a nonsteroidal antiinflammatory drug, such as flunixin meglumine, or a corticosteroid in nonpregnant animals.

Encouraging the animal to stand and walk and hydrotherapy of the affected limb may also be helpful.

Prevention of radial nerve paralysis consists of providing adequate footing for cattle and prevention of prolonged recumbency. Animals placed on tilt tables or in lateral recumbency for surgical procedures should have adequate shoulder and elbow padding, and prompt treatment should be instituted in animals recumbent secondary to metabolic disease.

In most cases of radial nerve paralysis secondary to traumatic ischemic injury, the animal recovers within several days.

BRACHIAL PLEXUS

The brachial plexus consists of 12 motor and sensory nerves originating from the C6-T2 nerve roots, providing complete innervation to the forelimb. Injury to the brachial plexus results in varying levels of damage to the radial, ulnar, and musculocutaneous nerves, with clinical signs dependent on severity of the lesion and nerves affected. Complete brachial plexopathy or brachial plexus avulsion results in complete motor and sensory deficits of the forelimb. It may be bilateral in cases of severe abduction of both forelimbs.

Brachial plexus paresis and paralysis has been reported in cattle secondary to trauma, inappropriate intramuscular injection, and compression secondary to neoplasia.[40,41] It may also result from lacerations, puncture wound, and infection of the axillary region.[42]

Diagnosis is based on clinical signs and history of trauma. Diagnosis may be confirmed and further characterized using electromyography.[40] Treatment consists of antiinflammatory therapy, splinting, and physical therapy. Complete avulsion of the brachial plexus carries a poor prognosis; however, limb amputation may be a reasonable option in small ruminants.

SUPRASCAPULAR NERVE

The suprascapular nerve originates from the C6-C7 nerve roots, innervating the supraspinatus and infraspinatus muscles. The primary function of these muscles is extension and lateral support of the shoulder joint. Damage to the suprascapular nerve is rare in cattle and is generally associated with trauma. Profound muscle atrophy of the supraspinatus and infraspinatus muscles is commonly noted. A case of suprascapular neuritis due to streptococcal meningoradiculitis in a cow has been reported.[43]

HIND LIMB

Hind limb peripheral nerve abnormalities in adult cattle are most commonly associated with calving trauma most often to the sciatic (peroneal branch) and obturator nerves. In calves, femoral nerve injury may be associated with forced extraction, particularly in calves in posterior presentation.

SCIATIC NERVE

Damage to this nerve or its associated branches (tibial and peroneal) is the most common peripheral nerve injury in cattle.[44] Damage to the peroneal nerve following prolonged dystocia can result in the calving paralysis syndrome seen most commonly in first calf heifers. The sciatic nerve arises from the L6-S2 nerve roots, innervating the extensors of the hip and hock and flexors of the stifle. The tibial branch of the sciatic nerve innervates the flexors of the fetlock, whereas the peroneal branch of the sciatic nerve innervates the extensors of the fetlock.

Clinical signs of sciatic nerve damage are variable and depend on the type of injury as well as the location of the injury. Most commonly, dropping of the hock and knuckling of the fetlock is seen, with weight bearing variable affected. Extension of the stifle should be maintained, as the femoral nerve controls it.

As previously mentioned, prolonged dystocia is a common cause of sciatic or peroneal nerve dysfunction. Damage to the tibial nerve on its own is uncommon. Other causes of sciatic nerve dysfunction include injection site abscesses or direct damage to the nerve during an intramuscular injection. The latter is more common in calves and small ruminants.

Treatment of sciatic nerve dysfunction includes bandaging to prevent abrasions of the fetlock and to encourage weight bearing. Recently, transposition of the vastus lateralis muscle has been described to treat peroneal nerve paralysis secondary to injection site lesions in calves.[45] Results of the study were promising; however, the applicability of the technique in adult cattle is not known at this time.

OBTURATOR NERVE INJURY

The obturator nerve arises from the L4-L6 nerve roots and is responsible for adduction of the pelvic limb. It is most commonly damaged secondary to compression following a prolonged dystocia; however, obturator nerve damage is less common than sciatic nerve damage following a dystocia.[46] Animals that become recumbent following calving or prolonged dystocia may have damage to both the obturator and sciatic nerves.[47]

In addition to damage secondary to calving, obturator damage may result from cattle slipping and abducting their hind limbs. Clinical signs of obturator nerve paralysis include an inability to adduct the limb, resulting in a splay-legged posture. Slippery footing can exacerbate the situation.

Treatment of obturator nerve paralysis consists of providing footing with excellent traction as well as hobbling the legs to prevent overabduction. Animals should be able to walk and bear weight normally once standing. Nonsteroidal antiinflammatory drugs or corticosteroids may be administered to decrease inflammation. If the animal is unable to bear weight, concurrent damage to the sciatic nerve, coxofemoral luxation, femoral fracture, or pelvic fracture should be considered.

FEMORAL NERVE

The femoral nerve arises from the L4-L6 nerve roots and is responsible for extension of the stifle and flexion of the hip. Damage to this nerve is seen most commonly in calves following forced extraction, particularly calves in a backwards presentation or calves that become hip locked.[48] It is thought to occur secondary to tearing due to overextension of the hip. In adult cattle, femoral nerve damage is uncommon but may occur secondary to the animal going down with the hind limbs retracted caudally, resulting in stretching or tearing of the nerve.

Animals with femoral nerve paralysis cannot support the affected limb because of a lack of extensor tone and take on a characteristic crouched posture if the injury is bilateral. Atrophy of the quadriceps femoris muscle may be noted 7 to 10 days after injury and patellar luxation may follow.

Treatment is similar to that for damage of other peripheral nerves, including antiinflammatory therapy and physiotherapy.[49] Use of a float tank may be beneficial in adult cattle, as these animals cannot bear weight on the affected limb.

GENETIC-ASSOCIATED NEUROLOGIC DISEASES

Several genetically determined neurologic diseases have been described in cattle affecting both the central nervous system and the peripheral nerves. These diseases include a familial neuropathy in Gelbvieh calves[50]; degenerative myeloencephalopathy of brown Swiss cattle (weaver syndrome)[51]; spinal muscle atrophy of Braunvieh, brown Swiss, Holstein-Friesian, and Red Danish[52–55]; degenerative axonopathy of Holstein-Friesian and Tyrolean Grey[56,57]; and progressive ataxia of Charolais.[58] These conditions are generally definitively diagnosed at postmortem examination.

REFERENCES

1. Braun U, Schweizer G, Gerspach C, et al. Clinical findings in 11 cattle with abscesses in the thoracic vertebrae. Vet Rec 2003;152:782–4.
2. Sherman DM, Ames TR. Vertebral body abscesses in cattle: a review of five cases. J Am Vet Med Assoc 1986;188:608–11.
3. Finley GG. A survey of vertebral abscesses in domestic animals in Ontario. Can Vet J 1975;16:114–7.
4. Stokol T, Divers TJ, Arrigan JW, et al. Cerebrospinal fluid findings in cattle with central nervous system disorders: a retrospective study of 102 cases (1990-2008). Vet Clin Pathol 2009;38:103–12.
5. Zani DD, Romano L, Scandella M, et al. Spinal epidural abscess in two calves. Vet Surg 2008;37:801–8.
6. Braun U, Dumelin J, Sydler T. Fracture of the lumbar vertebrae in two cows. Vet Rec 2007;160:162–3.
7. Edwards JF, Wikse SE, Loy JK, et al. Vertebral fracture associated with trauma during movement and restraint of cattle. J Am Vet Med Assoc 1995;207:934–5.
8. McDuffee LA, Ducharme NG, Ward JL. Repair of sacral fracture in two dairy cattle. J Am Vet Med Assoc 1993;202:1126–8.
9. Agerholm JS, Basse A, Arnbjerg J. Vertebral fractures in newborn calves. Acta Vet Scand 1993;34:379–84.
10. Schuijt G. Iatrogenic fractures of ribs and vertebrae during delivery in perinatally dying calves: 235 cases (1978-1988). J Am Vet Med Assoc 1990;197:1196–202.
11. Schuh JC, Killeen JR. A retrospective study of dystocia-related vertebral fractures in neonatal calves. Can Vet J 1988;29:830–3.
12. Frederick JD, Mackay RJ, Winter MD, et al. Vertebral osteomyelitis with abscessation in a Holstein calf. Vet Rec 2009;164:723–4.
13. Healy AM, Doherty ML, Monaghan ML, et al. Cervico-thoracic vertebral osteomyelitis in 14 calves. Vet J 1997;154:227–32.
14. Shupe JL, Butcher JE, Call JW, et al. Clinical signs and bone changes associated with phosphorus deficiency in beef cattle. Am J Vet Res 1988;49:1629–36.
15. Van Metre DC, Callan RJ, Garry FB. Examination of the musculoskeletal system in recumbent cattle. Compendium 2001;23(2):S5–24.
16. Gooneratne S, Buckley W, Christensen D. Review of copper deficiency and metabolism in ruminants. Can J Anim Sci 1989;69:819–45.
17. Hurlbert RJ, Hadley MN, Walters BC, et al. Pharmacological therapy for acute spinal cord injury. Neurosurgery 2013;72(Suppl 2):93–105.
18. Burton AJ, Nydam DV, Long ED, et al. Signalment and clinical complaints initiating hospital admission, methods of diagnosis, and pathological findings associated with bovine lymphosarcoma (112 cases). J Vet Intern Med 2010;24:960–4.

19. Marshak RR, Coriell LL, Lawrence WC, et al. Studies on bovine lymphosarcoma. I. Clinical aspects, pathological alterations, and herd studies. Cancer Res 1962; 22:202–17.

20. Meyer L. Wandering larvae of Hypoderma bovis in the spinal canal of young cattle. Dtsch Tierarztl Wochenschr 1973;80:397 [in German].

21. Hiepe T, Ribbeck R, Gahtow I, et al. Dynamics of infestation of cattle with Hypoderma bovis De Geer, 1776. 2. Occurrence of larvae I in the spinal canal and localization of the grubs in cattle. Monatsh Veterinarmed 1969;24:289–93 [in German].

22. Mitchell KJ, Peters-Kennedy J, Stokol T, et al. Diagnosis of Parelaphostrongylus spp. Infection as a cause of meningomyelitis in calves. J Vet Diagn Invest 2011;23:1097–103.

23. Dobey CL, Grunenwald C, Newman SJ, et al. Retrospective study of central nervous system lesions and association with Parelaphostrongylus species by histology and specific nested polymerase chain reaction in domestic camelids and wild ungulates. J Vet Diagn Invest 2014;26:748–54.

24. Guthery FS, Beasom SL, Jones L. Cerebrospinal nematodiasis caused by Parelaphostrongylus tenuis in Angora goats in Texas. J Wildl Dis 1979;15:37–42.

25. Rickard LG, Gentz EJ, Pearson EG, et al. Experimentally induced meningeal worm (Parelaphostrongylus tenuis) infection in the llama (Lama glama): clinical evaluation and implications for parasite translocation. J Zoo Wildl Med 1994; 25(3):390–402.

26. Culp WT, Ehrhart N, Withrow SJ, et al. Results of surgical excision and evaluation of factors associated with survival time in dogs with lingual neoplasia: 97 cases (1995-2008). J Am Vet Med Assoc 2013;242:1392–7.

27. Alden C, Woodson F, Mohan R, et al. Cerebrospinal nematodiasis in sheep. J Am Vet Med Assoc 1975;166:784.

28. Pybus MJ, Groom S, Samuel WM. Meningeal worm in experimentally-infected bighorn and domestic sheep. J Wildl Dis 1996;32:614–8.

29. Jortner BS, Troutt HF, Collins T, et al. Lesions of spinal cord parelaphostrongylosis in sheep. Sequential changes following intramedullary larval migration. Vet Pathol 1985;22:137–40.

30. Scarratt W, Karzenski S, Wallace M, et al. Suspected parelaphostrongylosis in five llamas. Progr Vet Neurol 1996;7:124–9.

31. Duncan RB Jr, Patton S. Naturally occurring cerebrospinal parelaphostrongylosis in a heifer. J Vet Diagn Invest 1998;10:287–91.

32. Pinn TL, Bender HS, Stokol T, et al. Cerebrospinal fluid eosinophilia is a sensitive and specific test for the diagnosis of Parelaphostrongylus tenuis in camelids in the northeastern United States. J Vet Diagn Invest 2013;25:54–60.

33. Nagy DW. Parelaphostrongylus tenuis and other parasitic diseases of the ruminant nervous system. Vet Clin North Am Food Anim Pract 2004;20:393–412, viii.

34. Alleyne T, Joseph J, Lalla A, et al. Cytochrome-c oxidase isolated from the brain of swayback-diseased sheep displays unusual structure and uncharacteristic kinetics. Mol Chem Neuropathol 1998;34:233–47.

35. Banton MI, Lozano-Alarcon F, Nicholson SS, et al. Enzootic ataxia in Louisiana goat kids. J Vet Diagn Invest 1990;2:70–3.

36. Coppock R, Mostrom M, Khan A, et al. A review of nonpesticide phosphate ester-induced neurotoxicity in cattle. Vet Hum Toxicol 1995;37:576–9.

37. Cho D, Leipold H. Spina bifida and spinal dysraphism in calves. Zentralbl Veterinarmed A 1977;24:680–95.

38. Hiraga T, Abe M. Anatomical observation of six calves affected with segmental aplasia of the spinal cord. Anat Rec 1987;219:402–8.
39. Doige C. Spina bifida in a calf. Can Vet J 1975;16:22.
40. Ruegsegger F, Steffen F, Nuss KA. Partial brachial plexus paresis in three calves. Vet Rec 2012;171:401.
41. Tremblay C, Girard C, Dubreuil P, et al. Synovial sarcoma in an Ayrshire heifer. Vet Pathol 2000;37:357–9.
42. Divers TJ. Acquired spinal cord and peripheral nerve disease. Vet Clin North Am Food Anim Pract 2004;20:231–42, v–vi.
43. Matsuda K, Sato N, Sakaguchi K, et al. Suprascapular nerve paralysis due to streptococcal meningoradiculitis in a cow. J Vet Med Sci 2008;70:1349–51.
44. Divers TJ, Rebhun WC, Peek SF. Rebhun's diseases of dairy cattle. 2nd edition. St Louis (MO): Saunders/Elsevier; 2007.
45. Kilic E, Yayla S, Aksoy O, et al. Treatment of peroneal paralysis with transposition of vastus lateralis muscle in calves. Vet Rec 2014;175:69.
46. Cox VS, Breazile JE, Hoover TR. Surgical and anatomic study of calving paralysis. Am J Vet Res 1975;36:427–30.
47. Levine JM, Levine GJ, Hoffman AG, et al. Comparative anatomy of the horse, ox, and dog: the vertebral column and peripheral nerves. Equine Comp Cont Educ Pract Vet 2007;2:279–92.
48. Tryphonas L, Hamilton GF, Rhodes CS. Perinatal femoral nerve degeneration and neurogenic atrophy of quadriceps femoris muscle in calves. J Am Vet Med Assoc 1974;164:801–7.
49. White AJ, White VJ. Physiotherapy as an aid to treatment of bilateral femoral paralysis in a calf. Vet Rec 1995;137:489–91.
50. Panciera R, Washburn K, Streeter R, et al. A familial peripheral neuropathy and glomerulopathy in Gelbvieh calves. Vet Pathol 2003;40:63–70.
51. Baird JD, Sarmiento UM, Basrur PK. Bovine progressive degenerative myeloencephalopathy (weaver syndrome) in brown Swiss cattle in Canada: a literature review and case report. Can Vet J 1988;29:370.
52. Dirksen G, Doll K, Hafner A, et al. Spinal muscle atrophy in brown Swiss x Braunvieh cross calves. Dtsch Tierarztl Wochenschr 1992;99:168–75 [in German].
53. Troyer D, Cash W, Vestweber J, et al. Review of spinal muscular atrophy (SMA) in Brown Swiss cattle. J Vet Diagn Invest 1993;5:303.
54. Pumarola M, Anor S, Majo N, et al. Spinal muscular atrophy in Holstein-Friesian calves. Acta Neuropathol 1997;93:178–83.
55. Agerholm J, Basse A. Spinal muscular atrophy in calves of the red Danish dairy breed. Vet Rec 1994;134:232–5.
56. Harper P, Healy P. Neurological disease associated with degenerative axonopathy of neonatal Holstein-Friesian calves. Aust Vet J 1989;66:143–6.
57. Drögemüller C, Reichart U, Seuberlich T, et al. An unusual splice defect in the mitofusin 2 gene (MFN2) is associated with degenerative axonopathy in Tyrolean Grey cattle. PLoS One 2011;6:e18931.
58. Cordy D. Progressive ataxia of Charolais cattle—an oligodendroglial dysplasia. Vet Pathol 1986;23:78–80.

Toxicoses of the Ruminant Nervous System

Gene A. Niles, DVM, MS

KEYWORDS

- Ruminant • Toxicosis • Polioencephalomalacia • Lead • Neurologic disease
- Infectious agents • Poisonous plants

KEY POINTS

- Damage to the nervous system of ruminants can be caused by organic compounds, inorganic compounds, metals, infectious agents, and plants.
- Specific agents that can cause damage include lead, salt, pesticides, insecticides, mountain laurel, nightshades, and milkweeds.
- Not all syndromes can be cured, and it is important that caution is used when using unapproved drugs to treat ruminant brain injuries.

INTRODUCTION

Numerous organic compounds, inorganic compounds, metals, infectious agents, and plants cause damage to the nervous system of ruminants. This article reviews many of these agents. This review is not meant to be exhaustive but rather a brief overview of the agent, its mechanism of action, clinical signs, diagnosis, and treatment of the most common neurotoxicoses encountered in ruminant medicine. Readers must use caution when using unapproved drugs to treat brain injuries to ruminants to avoid tissue residues.

NONINFECTIOUS AGENTS
Polioencephalomalacia

Polioencephalomalacia (PEM) is a diagnostic term describing necrosis of the gray matter of the brain. This lesion has become synonymous with the neurologic disease termed *polio*, which is documented in cattle, sheep, goats, cervids, camelids, and camels. Cerebrocortical necrosis and cortical laminar necrosis are synonymous with PEM. Historically, thiamine deficiency or destruction of thiamine by thiaminases, present in a variety of plants; by-products of rumen acidosis; and amprolium

Disclosure Statement: The author has nothing to disclose.
Rocky Ford Branch, Veterinary Diagnostic Laboratory System, Colorado State University, 24847 CR 21, Rocky Ford, CO 81067, USA
E-mail address: gene.niles@colostate.edu

administration were listed as the causes of this disease. Other causes of PEM include excess dietary sulfur, lead poisoning, and salt poisoning.

Excess dietary sulfur has been known to cause PEM for more than 30 years. Although numerous investigators have documented sulfur-induced PEM during this time period, the specific mechanism of action is open for debate. Historically the mechanism of action is thought to be that excess dietary sulfur leads to formation of excess hydrogen sulfide (H_2S), entering the bloodstream and causing direct damage to the brain. Rumen bacteria metabolize elemental, inorganic, and organic sulfur; therefore, the total sulfur content in feed and water must be determined to determine total sulfur intake.[1,2] These bacteria use sulfates for their own metabolic needs and the production of sulfur-containing amino acids releasing H_2S into the rumen.[1,2] It takes 7 days for these bacteria to acclimate to this process.[1–3] The H_2S accumulates in the rumen gas cap where it dissociates to HS^-, $HSO3^-$, S2, and S0. The amount of H_2S in the gas cap compared with the other ions is dependent on the rumen pH. When the rumen pH is 7.4, one-third is in the form of H_2S; this value increases to 97.2% when the rumen pH is 5.2. This explains why the incidence of PEM is much greater in animals fed concentrates. H_2S trapped in the rumen gas cap diffuses across the rumen wall entering into the portal blood stream. When large amounts of H_2S enter the blood, the liver's ability to convert it back to sulfate is overwhelmed, allowing direct access of excessive amounts of H_2S to the brain.

H_2S is produced endogenously and serves to protect the brain cells.[4] At normal physiologic levels it functions as a neuromodulator and protector of brain cells. It protects brain function by scavenging free radicals and reactive oxygen species, reducing oxidative stress and modulating glutathione and intracellular Ca^{2+} levels.[4] When excess amounts enter the brain, the added H_2S, HS^-, and $HSO3^-$ interfere with the electron transport chain by blocking cytochrome C, leading to cell death.[5–7] Damage occurs to the brain because of its high energy demand, with the greatest demand involving the gray matter due to the increased number of synapses compared with white matter.[8,9] Acute death due to respiratory failure can result from paralysis of the carotid body.[5,10,11]

Inhalation of eructated rumen gas is another proposed route of H_2S access into the blood. This route of entry is questioned by some investigators.[4,12,13] When expired air from weaned beef heifers receiving up to 7010 ppm sulfur in their ration and exhibiting clinical signs of PEM was analyzed for H_2S and other biomarkers indicative of oxidative lung damage, none was detected with repeated sampling. Also, histology did not reveal any lung damage in these animals when euthanized during episodes of clinical illness.[12] Other investigators question whether the amount of H_2S in rumen gas reaches amounts that are high enough to be significant even if appreciable amounts of eructated gas are inhaled.[4] This subject merits additional research to establish how H_2S enters the bloodstream.

Thiamine is a sulfur-containing water-soluble vitamin. It is synthesized in the stomach and intestines of all animals but nonruminants require additional dietary sources. Rumen bacteria are capable of synthesizing adequate amounts of thiamine even with less than optimal nutrition.[14]

Thiamine monophosphate (TMP) and thiamine pyrophosphate (TPP) are phosphate esters of thiamine that are essential for normal metabolism. TPP is an essential coenzyme in 6 different decarboxylation reactions in aerobic respiration.[6,15] This coenzyme is the catalyst to convert pyruvate to acetyl coenzyme A, which reacts with oxaloacetate in the citric acid cycle in aerobic respiration.[15] Thiamine is essential for normal cellular membrane function and the conduction of nerve impulses.[6] Because of the high energy demands of the central nervous system (CNS), adequate thiamine is important to maintain CNS health. This is one explanation as to why supplemental thiamine benefits patients with CNS disease. Increased dietary thiamine has been shown to decrease the severity of clinical signs of PEM even when microscopic brain lesions were present.[16]

Other theories as to the mechanism of action of excess sulfur propose that there is a direct interaction between thiamine and sulfur that interferes with the function of thiamine itself or TMP and TPP instead of a direct action of the sulfur radicals on nerve cells.[4,17] Another proposal is that increased dietary sulfur increases the demand for TPP, which is necessary to carry on normal metabolism within the brain.[4] Readers are directed to the articles published by Amat and colleagues for further discussion concerning these proposed mechanisms of action.

Sources of increased sulfur include feed containing by-products of the grain, dairy, and sugar industries, which are known to contain high sulfur levels. Water sources containing high sulfate levels are found in the Great Plains and throughout the inter-mountain regions of the United States and Canada and have caused PEM either by themselves or in conjunction with sulfur-accumulating plants, such as kochia and this-tles. Polio has occurred in ruminants grazing small grain pastures fertilized with sulfate fertilizers and in animals exposed to H_2S pit gases and elemental sulfur.[17]

Two syndromes occur with PEM. In one syndrome, signs occur acutely, and the animals are found dead or recumbent and comatose. These animals generally have irreparable brain damage and fail to respond to treatment. Euthanasia should be considered if the animal does not show a rapid response to treatment.

Clinical signs associated with the second syndrome vary depending on length of exposure and degrees of CNS impairment. Early signs include ataxia, fine muscle tremor of the head and face, nervousness, belligerence, teeth grinding, salivation, circling, head pressing, cortical blindness, and stupor. The blindness is characterized by the lack of a menace reflex whereas the palpebral reflex remains intact and the pupils respond to light. Nystagmus with medial-dorsal strabismus (stargazing) may occur. If the disease progresses, additional clinical signs include lateral recumbency and opisthotonus; clonic-tonic convulsions with paddling motion and death occur. Some recovered animals, known as *brainers*, are unproductive due to permanent brain damage. These animals should be salvaged, when applicable.[11] Exposure to H_2S from manure pits can cause paralysis of the carotid body with acute death due to respiratory failure.[5,10]

Treatment of PEM is symptomatic. When animals with minimal clinical signs of CNS impairment are ambulatory and eating, removal from the source results in recovery in most animals.[18] Therapy includes thiamine administered at 10 mg/kg to 20 mg/kg intravenously (IV) or intramuscularly 2 to 3 times the first day followed by the same dose twice a day for 2 to 3 more days. Dexamethasone, at 1 mg/kg to 2 mg/kg, aids in reduction of cerebral edema. Mannitol, furosemide, dimethyl sulfoxide, sedatives, and tranquilizers may be used to control seizures, when applicable.

Lesions associated with PEM include herniation of the cerebellum into the magnum foramen resulting from brain swelling and edema. The brain may become soft due to loss of turgidity and tone and spongy in texture. Flattening of the cerebral gyri with yellow-brown discoloration may occur. Bilateral laminar cortical malacia may be visible and fluoresce under ultraviolet light. Hemorrhage and cavitation of the cerebral laminae can occur.[19]

Microscopic lesions include small or absent neurons in the affected areas. Astrocytes become acidophilic and swollen and lose their processes, creating increased space between neurons. Spongiform degeneration is indicated by eosinophilic globules filling the space of the dead neurons. An increase in the size of the blood vessels and macrophage density occurs. Healing is evidenced by the presence of astrogliosis.[19]

Diagnosis of sulfur-induced PEM is made by the presence of PEM lesions coupled with a history of consumption of feed, plants, or water containing high amounts of sulfur. Measurement of rumen H_2S in animals exhibiting clinical PEM is usually of no value because H_2S levels rapidly decline as animal go off feed.[12] Research is ongoing concerning measurement of rumen H_2S and urine thiosulfate in herd mates to assess sulfur exposure levels in groups of cattle.[20]

The effects of sulfur are additive; therefore, total sulfur intake from feed and water must be determined to determine total sulfur intake. A program to calculate total sulfur intake can be found at the following Web site: http://dlab.colostate.edu/webdocs/tools/sulfurcalc.cfm. The National Research Council recommends that the maximum tolerable level of sulfur in cattle is 0.3% for animals fed greater than 85% concentrates and 0.5% for animals consuming greater than 40% forage.[21]

Lead

Poisoning occurs most often in cattle due to their inquisitive nature.[22–26] Exposure to lead batteries and lead-based paints are the most common sources of lead. Lead batteries have been baled into hay and ground into mixed feeds. Exposure to lead-contaminated pastures is the most common route of exposure for sheep.[26] Other sources include lead-based lubricants, joint compounds, putty and caulking material, solder, roofing felt, linoleum, and lead shot.[26] Lead poisoning is most common in young animals, which absorb up to 50% of the lead they ingest, whereas older animals absorb 1% to 3% of ingested lead.[24] Lead affects animals by binding sulfhydryl groups, which inactive enzymes, interfere with vitamin D metabolism, and compete with calcium ions.[23,26] The majority of ingested lead is eliminated unchanged in the feces. Absorbed lead is eliminated in urine and milk. Retention of lead particles in the rumen and reticulum prolong the elimination of lead in ruminants with a half-life of 135 days (range 3–577 days).[24] Bishoff and colleagues[24] reported that 4% to 12% of the animals in herds with clinical lead poisoning were asymptomatic but had blood lead levels of greater than 0.35 ppm, which is consistent with acute poisoning. Lead exposure to ruminants poses a risk to humans due to consumption of meat and milk and is reportable in some states; animals with blood lead levels of greater than or equal to 0.05 ppm are quarantined.[23] To reduce risk to humans, testing of samples of whole blood from all animals in a herd exposed to lead is recommended.

Clinical signs observed with lead poisoning range from acute death to typical signs seen with PEM. Animals that die acutely may not exhibit any postmortem lesions whereas lesions typical of PEM may occur in animals showing clinical disease. Red blood cells contain greater than 90% of the lead; therefore, diagnosis of lead poisoning in live animals requires submission of whole blood preserved in anticoagulant tubes. Blood lead levels greater than 0.35 ppm confirm a diagnosis of lead poisoning. Liver and kidney lead levels greater than or equal to 10 ppm in either tissue confirm a postmortem diagnosis of lead poisoning. In the author's experience, gross and microscopic lesions are generally lacking with lead poisoning. The rumen and reticulum should be inspected for lead particles. Microscopic lesions of cerebellar laminar necrosis occur occasionally. Rarely, eosinophilic meningitis is noted microscopically with lead poisoning.[27]

Calcium disodium EDTA (CaEDTA) (60–110 mg/kg), administered IV or subcutaneously in divided doses for up to 5 days, and thiamine (2–5 mg/kg) are used to treat lead poisoning.[28–30] The use of British anti-Lewisite or penicillamine to chelate lead is reported to be less effective in the treatment of lead poisoning in cattle than CaEDTA alone.[29] Zinc and other divalent trace mineral levels should be monitored when CaEDTA is given for prolonged periods of time. Experimentally, succimer (meso-2-3-dimercaptosuccinic acid) has been shown more effective than CaEDTA in treating calves with lead poisoning.[31] Administration of magnesium sulfate laxatives forms insoluble lead salts, which decrease rumen absorption. Rumenotomy may be needed to remove large lead particles. Supportive care including the use of tranquilizers to control seizures may be necessary.

Salt

Salt poisoning is also known as water deprivation–sodium ion toxicosis. Acute or direct sodium ion toxicosis stems from consumption of excess salt in livestock feed or high saline water and generally manifests with clinical signs of acute gastrointestinal disease. Formulations of milk replacers that contain excess salt and incorrect mixing of milk replacers or electrolyte solutions are other causes of sodium ion toxicosis in bottle fed calves.[32] Acute deaths can occur when salt-starved animals are allowed access to unlimited salt supplements. Neurologic signs can follow acute illness. More commonly, indirect toxicosis results from restricted water intake over a period of several days. Clinical signs compatible with PEM are seen after these animals are allowed unlimited access to water. Reasons for water deprivation are numerous, including frozen water sources, unpalatable water sources, overcrowding, malfunction of automatic waterers, and neglect.

Acute hypernatremia occurs when serum sodium levels reach 160 mEq/L within 24 to 48 hours. When this occurs, cell integrity is maintained by rapidly accumulating sodium and other electrolytes within the brain neurons to equalize the osmotic pressure and prevent fluid loss. If the hypernatremia is quickly resolved without neuron damage, the electrolyte levels within the brain cells decline in accordance with the decline of sodium in the cerebrospinal fluid (CSF). With prolonged hyponatremia, organic molecules called idiogenic solutes enter the brain cells, increasing the osmolality to aid in preventing water loss and cell shrinkage. When this mechanism fails, the neurons dehydrate and shrink, resulting in hemorrhage, brain infarcts, and edema. This damage interferes with the production of energy via glycolysis, which limits the energy available for normal function. Sodium passively enters the CSF but requires energy to be transported out of the CSF. In sodium ion toxicosis, sodium is trapped in the CSF and brain due to the lack of available energy for active transport out of the CSF. If access to unlimited water occurs and the animal rehydrates, an osmotic gradient is established between the blood and CSF, resulting in an influx of fluid into the CSF. The resultant cerebral edema causes the clinical signs of PEM.

Normal reference ranges for sodium in serum and CSF are 135 mEq/L to 155 mEq/L and 135 mEq/L to 150 mEq/L, respectively. Serum levels of greater than 160 mEq/L confirm a diagnosis of hypernatremia. CSF fluid samples should be analyzed in suspect animals that have normal serum sodium values. In addition to CSF sodium levels, brain, rumen content, and ocular fluid are beneficial in establishing a postmortem diagnosis. The normal range for sodium in the brain of cattle is 1600 ppm to 1800 ppm. Brain sodium levels greater than 1800 ppm and rumen levels of greater than 9000 ppm support a diagnosis of sodium ion toxicosis.[29,33] Normal values for brain sodium are lacking in other ruminants. The sodium content in ocular fluid can be used to assess sodium values for up to 48 hours postmortem.[34] Aqueous and vitreous humor sodium levels have essentially equal values for up to 24 hours postmortem; therefore, either value can be used to evaluate postmortem sodium levels within 24 hours of death. The normal value for sodium in vitreous humor is equal to 95% of the serum value.[35]

Treatment of sodium ion toxicosis is generally unrewarding, with greater than or equal to 50% mortality. Rehydration of hypernatremic animals should be done slowly to prevent iatrogenic cerebral edema. Ideally, this should be accomplished over a 48-hour to 72-hour time period. On a herd basis, water should be limited to 0.5% of body weight at 60-minute intervals until the animals are rehydrated. When applicable in treating individual animals, the serum sodium should be determined and the sodium level should not be reduced by more than 0.3 mEq/h to 0.5 mEq/h.[36] Administration of hypertonic saline solutions closely matching the serum sodium levels is recommended to prevent osmotic gradients that cause increased cerebral edema.[36,37] When the serum sodium level is not known, solutions containing 170 mEq/L of sodium can be used initially and gradually reduced as the clinical signs improve. Successful treatment of hypernatremic scouring calves using 5% dextrose and isotonic sodium bicarbonate has been reported. Although this therapy reduced the serum sodium concentrations 4 times faster than recommended, calves recovered uneventfully.[38] When clinical signs of cerebral edema are evident, administration of dexamethasone, mannitol, and dimethyl sulfoxide to reduce brain swelling and sedatives to control seizures may be beneficial. Care should be taken to avoid tissue residues of drugs that are not approved for use in food animals.

Bovine Bonkers

Bovine hysteria and ammoniated feed syndrome are names for this neurologic disease with clinical signs of nervousness and hyperexcitability followed by mania that occurs in cattle and sheep. When the animals are startled they may stampede into objects and fences, as if blind. Nervousness, ear twitching, trembling, jaw champing, salivation, frequent urination and defecation, and convulsions can occur. Generally, animals seem normal when left alone for 15 to 20 minutes. Repeated stimuli initiate the cycle again. The toxin involved is 4-methylimidazole, which is found in ammoniated forages, molasses products, and protein blocks. The toxin is eliminated in milk, causing disease in nursing calves and lambs. Rapid removal from the source generally results in rapid recovery. Death may occur due to trauma.

Urea Toxicosis

Urea toxicosis has been reported in cattle, sheep, and goats fed protein supplements containing nonprotein nitrogen (NPN) products.[39,40] Urea is the major NPN source added to ruminant feeds. Ureases in the rumen convert the NPN to ammonia (NH_3), which is used by the rumen bacteria to synthesize amino acids and utilizable proteins. This process takes energy requiring readily available carbohydrates. It takes 5 to 7 days for the rumen microflora to acclimate to efficient use of NPN but this acclimation is lost in as little as 1 day. Urea toxicosis occurs when unacclimated cattle gain access to feeds containing NPN. Toxicosis also occurs when acclimated animals are fed excess amounts of NPN products or animals consume fertilizers containing NPN. When the rumen pH is neutral to acidic, unutilized NH_3 is converted to ammonium, which remains in the rumen. Toxicosis occurs when the production of NH_3 outpaces the ability of the rumen bacteria to convert it to utilizable proteins. The increasing amount of NH_3 increases the rumen pH to greater than or equal to 8, allowing excess NH_3 to accumulate in the rumen. The NH_3 is absorbed into the blood and disrupts the tricarboxylic acid (TCA) cycle. Clinical signs occur in as little as 20 minutes in cattle and 30 minutes in sheep.[39] Tremors, muscular weakness, dyspnea, increased urination and defecation, and convulsions occur. Many animals are found dead. Blood samples from live animals require immediate analysis for NH_3, which is impractical in general practice. Postmortem samples include rumen content, CSF, and ocular fluid, which should be frozen within 1 hour and kept frozen until they arrive at the laboratory. Normal blood, serum, ocular fluid, and CNS NH_3 values are less than 0.5 mg/dL. Clinical signs occur at approximately 1 mg/dL and death at 3 mg/dL. Because of the volatility of NH_3, agreement of 3 or more of the samples is needed to support a diagnosis of NPN toxicosis.[39] Treatment of urea toxicosis includes administration of cold water (20–40 L) to slow down the metabolism of the rumen microbes and 5% acetic acid (0.5–2 L sheep; 4–8 L cattle), to decrease rumen pH. For prevention, ruminants should be slowly acclimated to NPN and given feeds that supply adequate energy to use the NPN. Urea should not constitute more than one-third of the total nitrogen in the ration. The amount of the urea should be less than 3% of the concentrate portion of the ration and not exceed 1% of the total ration. Raw soybeans contain urease and should not be fed to animals consuming NPN.

Organophosphorus

Organophosphorus (OP) and carbamate pesticides are used throughout agriculture and the general public. They contain some of the most dangerous chemicals known to humans. Ruminants are exposed to these pesticides by sprays, topical application, and oral administration. They are readily absorbed by all routes. Carbamate and OP pesticides block the action of acetylcholinesterase (AChE), resulting in the accumulation of acetylcholine at cholinergic and neuromuscular nerve junctions, resulting in repetitive firing of the parasympathetic nervous system. OP compounds form an irreversible bond with AChE, whereas the bond formed with carbamates is reversible, allowing it to spontaneously dislodge.[41] Clinical signs of salivation, lacrimation, urination, and defecation (SLUD) occur within minutes or possibly as long as 12 hours after exposure. Muscle tremors, dyspnea, bloat, coma, seizures, and death occur. Administration of atropine or pralidoxime is used to treat OP toxicosis. Pralidoxime is not indicated for the treatment of carbamate toxicosis because the bond between AChE and carbamate pesticides reverses spontaneously.[41] Administration of activated charcoal is indicated to absorb ingested toxins and animals should be thoroughly bathed with dish soap in cases of topical application. Diagnosis of OP toxicosis is accomplished by measurement of AChE in samples of whole blood in live animals and samples of retina and brain postmortem. Because the bond between carbamates and AChE reverses spontaneously, measurement of blood AChE is not a reliable indicator of carbamate exposure. Postmortem analysis for carbamate and OP compounds in whole blood, rumen content, liver, and fat can be used to confirm exposure.

Organophosphorus-Induced Polyneuropathy

OP-induced polyneuropathy, or dying-back syndrome, is a delayed or chronic neurotoxic syndrome. It can occur 10 days to a few months after exposure to OP compounds containing triorthocresyl phosphate, which is found in lubricants, hydraulic oil, and solvents.[41–44] To a lesser extent, commonly used OP insecticides have caused delayed polyneuropathy in animals and humans.[45] Inhibition of the neuropathy target esterase is thought to be the mechanism of action for this delayed response.[41,45] Posterior weakness and ataxia occur anywhere from 1 week to 3 months after exposure. Paralysis with loss of tone to the tail, anus, and bladder follows. There is no treatment of this syndrome. Microscopic evidence of axonal degeneration aids diagnosis. Fat biopsies can be analyzed for OP residues to help establish exposure.

Organochlorine

Organochlorine (OC) insecticides have not been used in agriculture for many years due to their persistence in the environment. Although banned from use, OC toxicosis periodically occurs today. Poisoning usually occurs when animals break into sheds and out-buildings on old homesteads and farms where these products were stored for years. Clinical signs observed with OC toxicosis are hypersensitivity, nervousness, twitching of the facial muscles followed by spasms of the neck and hindquarters, and convulsions. Treatment includes activated charcoal to promote elimination and symptomatic therapy to control seizures. OCs accumulate in fat and are eliminated in milk. Laboratory analysis of rumen content, fat and milk are used to confirm exposure.[46]

Cyanobacteria

Cyanobacteria (blue-green algae) blooms typically occur on stagnant bodies of water with high nutrient content when temperatures exceed 20°C. Runoff from fields fertilized with nitrogen and phosphorus fertilizers greatly potentiate the occurrence of algae blooms. Species of *Anabaena*, *Oscillatoria*, and *Planktothrix* produce anatoxin-a. Anatoxin-as is produced by *Anabaena* spp.[47] Anatoxin-a depolarizes nicotinic receptors leading to rapid death due to respiratory paralysis. Anatoxin-as blocks AChE, producing clinical signs similar to organic phosphate poisoning. Death from either of these toxins can occur within minutes. Clinical signs include tremors, salivation, diarrhea, rigidity, and convulsions. Treatment of anatoxin-a is symptomatic to control seizures. Atropine is used to treat anatoxin-as.[48] Diagnosis is based on laboratory analysis of rumen content and water sources by chemical and microscopic analysis.

Strychnine

Strychnine is commonly found in mole and gopher baits. Strychnine works at the level of the spinal cord by inhibiting the action of glycine, which is manifested by extreme muscle rigidity and tetanic convulsions. Loud noises can lead to muscle spasms followed by opisthotonos, arched back, and extensor rigidity. Treatment includes reducing noise, controlling seizures, and administration of activated charcoal and laxatives, when applicable. Strychnine can be detected in blood and urine. Postmortem examination of rumen content for grain dyed red or green and laboratory analysis of rumen content or urine for strychnine give the best chance for detection.[49]

Zinc and Aluminum Phosphide

Zinc phosphide is used to control rodents and gophers. Aluminum phosphide is used to control weevils in stored grain. These compounds are stable when dry. When moistened or in contact with an acid, phosphine gas (PH_3) is liberated. PH_3 smells like acetylene or rotten fish and is heavier than air. It is thought to disrupt oxidative phosphorylation in mitochondria by inhibiting cytochrome C oxidase.[50] Furthermore, it increases reactive oxygen species, causing other oxidative cell damage.[51] Toxicosis generally occurs when these products have been used to control pests in stored feeds and are not allowed sufficient time for the PH_3 to dissipate before being fed. Bins of treated feed should be ventilated after the recommended 7-day treatment period and not fed for at least 10 days from the time of treatment.[50] Clinical signs can occur within minutes of exposure with death in a few hours. Although nonspecific, weakness, ataxia, hyperesthesia, recumbency, and seizures may be observed.[51] Therapy involves administration of magnesium sulfate laxatives with activated charcoal and 5% sodium bicarbonate to increase the rumen pH, slowing the release of PH_3, and supportive care to treat acidosis and shock. Laboratory diagnosis involves detection of PH_3 in rumen content or feed that has been packaged in airtight containers. Analysis of tissue samples for elevated zinc or aluminum levels may aid in a diagnosis.

When dealing with suspected PH_3 toxicosis, caution should be taken to avoid exposure to PH_3 gas present in the samples or carcass.[50]

Metaldehyde

Metaldehyde is used as a slug and snail bait. Cases of toxicosis occur primarily in coastal areas. Its mechanism of action is not fully understood but decreases in brain neurotransmitters and γ-aminobutyric acid (GABA) are documented. Clinical signs include tremors, ataxia, nystagmus, blindness, loss of menace reflex, salivation, and convulsions. Treatment involves administration of activated charcoal and mineral oil and symptomatic therapy to control seizures. Rumen content, serum, plasma, and urine should be frozen immediately and submitted for laboratory analysis.[52]

INFECTIOUS AGENTS
Botulism

Botulism is caused by neurotoxins found in *Clostridium botulinum*, *C barati*, and *C butyricum*.[53] Of the 8 antigenic groups or types (A–G) that cause illness, groups C and D are the ones most often associated with ruminant disease.[53] Contamination of hay, silage, and small grain forage preserved in plastic tubes or bags by type C botulism and feeding of poultry litter containing types C and D are the most common routes of exposure to ruminants. In Europe, the mosaic variant C/D is a common cause of botulism in cattle.[54] It has been proposed that broilers are subclinical carriers of *C botulinum* type D.[55] Less commonly, ruminants are affected by type B botulism from consuming hay contaminated with type B spores.[56] Botulinum toxins block the release of acetylcholine at the neuromuscular junction resulting in progressive flaccid paralysis. Loss of muscle tone to the tongue and tail and inability to urinate and defecate are signs of botulism. The tongue test assesses the ability of the animal to control tongue movements. Inability of an animal to resist or retract its tongue when pulled laterally from the mouth is characteristic of botulism. Manual movement of the jaws from side to side without resistance further supports the diagnosis.

In Germany, France, the Netherlands, and the United Kingdom, there are reports of a chronic form of botulism known as visceral botulism that affects cattle and humans.[57] In cattle, digestive upsets; laminitis; edema of the legs, udder, and brisket; dyspnea; and acute death occur. In adult humans who have close contact with cattle, dizziness, blurred vision, nausea, and difficulty speaking, breathing, and swallowing occur.[57]

Cattle are much more sensitive to botulism than mice, making the use of the mouse bioassay to diagnose botulism generally unrewarding.[55] Polymerase chain reaction and ELISA techniques can detect botulism toxins but are not routinely available, at this time.[58,59] When diagnosed, the source of the toxin should be removed and individual animals treated symptomatically. Although effective multivalent vaccines against type C and D botulism are used in other countries, none is licensed for use in the United States.[60] Botulism involving lactating dairy cattle poses a public health risk, especially to people consuming raw milk products.[61] Botulism toxin is listed as a category A agent by the Centers for Disease Control and Prevention, posing a high risk to the general public.[62] Standard pasteurization of milk has been shown to inactivate 99.99% of botulism toxins due to types A and B.[62]

Tetanus

Tetanus occurs when *C tetani* organisms gain entry into a susceptible animal and undergo anaerobic growth. Wounds, surgical sites, postcalving uterine infections, shearing, castration, and tail docking are common sites of infection. The use of elastrator bands in sheep, goats, and cattle promote the incidences of clinical cases of tetanus when preventative measures are not used. Tetanolysin and tetanospasmin are toxins produced by *C tetani*. Tetanolysin causes necrosis at the site of infection, promoting anaerobic growth of *C tetani*. Clinical disease is caused by tetanospasmin, which is transported through motor neuron axons to the spinal cord, where it irreversibly binds with Renshaw cells, preventing the release of GABA, which inhibits motor nerve function.[63,64] The lack of inhibition results in muscle spasms characteristic of tetanus.[64] Muscle rigidity, generalized stiffness, prolapse of the third lid when startled, sawhorse stance, stiff-legged gait, erect ears, rigid elevated tail head, and inability to open mouth (locked jaw) occur with tetanus. Recumbency with tetanic, stiff-legged seizures occurs terminally. Diagnosis is based on clinical signs coupled with a history of previous wounds, surgery, or parturition. Postmortem diagnosis is difficult because there are no specific gross or microscopic lesions. When possible, isolation of *C tetani* from infected wounds or surgical sites aids in diagnosis. The prognosis for ruminants with tetanus is poor. Penicillin, tetanus antitoxin, and medication to control muscle spasms along with supportive care are used to treat animals with tetanus. In situations where tetanus is prevalent, vaccination with tetanus toxoid beforehand or giving tetanus antitoxin at the time surgical procedures are performed is indicated.

Clostridium perfringens Type D

C perfringens type D produces epsilon toxin, resulting in sudden death in lambs, kids, and calves. Sudden death syndrome, also known as overeating or pulpy kidney disease, affects animals from a few weeks old up to 10 months. The toxin targets the brain, causing liquefactive necrosis, edema, and hemorrhage.[65] Sudden death of well-nourished, growing animals is the most common finding. Incoordination, trembling, and convulsions may be seen, with death occurring in 30 to 90 minutes.[66] Diagnosis is generally based on the clinical history. The presence of glycosuria supports the diagnosis. The postmortem findings of large swollen kidneys (pulpy kidney) due to rapid decomposition is variable. Administration of type D antitoxin is beneficial, if given at the first signs of illness, and is used for prevention of disease during outbreaks. When applicable, administration of *C perfringens* type D vaccine offers greater protection. Although not licensed for goats, routine use is common but some vaccines are not effective in goats.[67]

Neurotoxic Plants

Table 1 lists plants that cause clinical signs of nervous system disease. Only a few of these plants, such as the endophyte-infected pasture grasses, water hemlock, larkspurs, and a few others, are palatable to ruminants, when green. Livestock that have available, palatable forage generally avoid most poisonous plants unless they are forced to eat them because of mismanagement, overgrazing, or drought. Animals may eat toxic plants that remain green in the winter or turn green earlier than other forages. The palatability of some plants increases when dry and they are readily eaten in hay. Application of herbicides, such as 2,4-dichlorophenoxyacetic acid, to eliminate plants, such as jimsonweed, can increase their palatability, resulting in toxicosis.

Some species of poisonous plants, such as kochia and *Astragalus* sp, are heavily relied on for livestock feed and only sporadically cause illness. Ingestion of toxic plants, such as *Astragalus*, can be a learned behavior with animals becoming habituated to the plant.[66] Habituated animals seek it out even when moved to pastures with abundant palatable forage available.

Table 1
Neurotoxic plants of ruminants

Plant	Common Name	Toxin; Mechanism of Action	Species Affected	Time from Exposure to Onset of Clinical Signs	Clinical Signs	Notes
Worldwide						
Kalmia *Rhododendron* *Leucothoe*	Mountain laurel Azaleas Andromeda peris, eubotry, lyonia peris, ledum	Granotoxins; block sodium channels	Sheep Goats Cattle Camelid	Weeks	Respiratory depression bradycardia, profuse salivation, nasal discharges, bloat, abdominal pain, impaired vision, seizures	Unpalatable: green in winter, garden trimmings human toxicosis—"mad honey" bees also die from the toxin
Throughout United States						
Cicuta maculata	Water hemlock, spotted cowbane	Cicutoxin; suspected GABA inhibition, sodium and/or potassium channel blocker	All livestock	Within minutes	Muscle twitching: lips, ears, nose, and face; jaw chomping; teeth grinding; tongue lacerations; bloat; violent seizures	Palatable, remains toxic in hay
Conium maculatum	Poison hemlock	Pyridine alkaloids; coniine, N-methylconiine, γ-coniceine Low dose; block spinal reflexes High dose; nondepolarizing neuromuscular blockade	Cattle Sheep Goats Elk	Hours	Incoordination tremors, weakness, salivation, lacrimation, excitement followed by depression, progressive paresis, and death several hours later	Rare highly unpalatable when mature; contamination of hay fields, green chop

(continued on next page)

Table 1
(continued)

Plant	Common Name	Toxin; Mechanism of Action	Species Affected	Time from Exposure to Onset of Clinical Signs	Clinical Signs	Notes
Kochia scoparia	Burning bush, Mexican fire-weed	High sulfur content PEM	Cattle Sheep Goats	Several days	Muscle tremors, circling, blindness, ataxia, head pressing, bruxism, belligerence, depression	Heavily relied on for cattle feed in southwest US additive with high sulfate water
Dicentra cicullaria	Dutchman's breeches, little staggerweed	Isoquinolone alkaloids: cularidine; dopamine antagonist	Cattle Sheep	Requires consumption of 1.6% body weight	Periodic episodes of trembling, ropey salivation, ataxia, and possible seizures lasting <30 min, rapid recovery	Rare: palatable rich moist soils along stream banks
Equisetum arvense	Common horsetail	Unknown	Cattle	Requires ingestion of large amounts of green forage	Diarrhea, ataxia, loss of equilibrium, belligerence, seizures	Rare; wet areas
Lathyrus sylvestris *L latiolius*	Flat pea, caley pea, everlasting pea	Novel amino acids: ODAP[1], DABA[2], OxDABA[3]; presumed to antagonize central glutamate kainate quisqualate receptors	Sheep Cattle	Disease results after prolonged ingestion of a large amount of forage	Sheep: depression, anorexia, ataxia, circling, head pressing, bruxism, sawhorse stance, seizures, few die cattle: similar to sheep but generally transient with recovery in a few days	Ingestion of developing seeds while in the legumes [1]β-N-oxalyl-amino-αβ-diamino-propionic acid [2]α,γ-dia-amino butyric acid [3]γ-N-oxalyl-ι-α, γ-diaminobutyric acid

		Toxin	Species	Acute	Clinical signs	
Vicia villosa	Hairy vetch	Cyanogenic glycosides: γ-L-glutamyl-β-cyano-L-alanine	Cattle	Acute	Bellowing, seizures, sudden, death	Clinical signs mimic rabies, consumption of seeds
Zigadenus nuttallii *Z veneosus* *Z paniculatus*	Death camas Meadow death camas Sheathed death camas	Cervine-type veratrum Alkaloids: germine, protoverine, zygademine	Sheep Cattle	<24 h	Sheep: profuse ropey salivation, severe depression hyperexcitable, ataxia, trembling, arched back, stiff-legged, hopping gait, coma, death	Greatest risk early spring Cattle: profuse ropey salivation, depression, bruxism, recovery in 1–2 d
Delphinium sp	Larkspur	Diterpene alkaloids; inhibits acetylcholine at nicotinic sites, neuromuscular blockade	Cattle Sheep (low risk)	3–4 h	Tremors, ataxia, wide stance, stiff gait, fall repeatedly and cannot rise, recumbency, death	Primarily the western mountains, primary risk at flowering when palatable and toxin increases
Solanum sp	Nightshades	Glycolalkaloids, solanidines; tropane alkaloids,	Cattle Goats	Days	Depression, anorexia, apoxia, weakness	Substantial amounts must be eaten
Solanum dimidiatum	Western horse nettle, crazy cow syndrome	calystegins; inhibits α-mannosidase	Cattle	Weeks	Crazy cow syndrome: abrupt tremors, incoordination and collapse occurs following abrupt stimulation able to stand after brief rest	Crazy cow syndrome—central Texas
Zamia integrifolia	Palm	Glycosides of methyl-azoxy-methanol, β-N-methyl-amino-L-alanine	Cattle	Weeks	Progressive posterior weakness, stumbling, ataxia, and occasional goose-stepping	Ingestion of leaves

(continued on next page)

Table 1
(continued)

Plant	Common Name	Toxin; Mechanism of Action	Species Affected	Time from Exposure to Onset of Clinical Signs	Clinical Signs	Notes
Robinia pseudoacacia	Black locust	Unknown Robinin Robitin	Cattle Sheep Goats	Rapid onset	Belligerence, weakness, mydriasis, posterior ataxia,	Rare; ingestion of bark
Agrostema githago	Corn cockle	Steroidal Saponins	Cattle	Hours to days	Anorexia, bloat, diarrhea, salivation, tremors, paralysis	Contamination of grain and hay
Helenium sp, *Hymenoxys* sp Pingue	Sneezeweed, rubberweed, spewing disease	Pseudoguainolide Sesquiterpene Lactones	Sheep Goats Cattle	Weeks; rarely acute disease can occur within 4 h	Anorexia, ataxia, arched back, bruxism, muscle tremors, head pressing, regurgitation of foamy green saliva	Effects are cumulative
Solidago spectabilus S flexicaulis	Western goldenrod Broad leaved goldenrod	Unknown	Sheep	Hours	Excess salivation, constant lip and jaw movement, muscle tremors spread from head progressing over body, ataxia, seizures	Toxic in hay
Descurania pinnata	Tansy mustard	High sulfur content PEM	Cattle	Days	Anorexia, blindness, circling, tongue paralysis, weakness, tremors	Additive with high sulfate water
Atriplex Kochia Salicornia Sarcobatus	Saltbrush Burning bush Glasswort Greasewood	High sulfur content PEM	Cattle Sheep	Days	Anorexia, ataxia, blindness, circling, weakness, tremors	Additive with high sulfate water

Northern United States

Trifolium pratense	Red clover	Slaframine	Cattle Sheep	Days	Excessive stringy saliva, lacrimation, diarrhea, stiffness	Fungal endophyte: *Rhizoctonia legumeinicola*
Ranunculus acris *R bulbosus*	Tall buttercup bulbous buttercup	Ranunculin	Sheep Cattle	Days	Tremors, weakness, seizures, paralysis, depression, watery diarrhea, dyspnea	Rare substantial amounts must be eaten

Southern United Sstates

Acacia berlandieri	Guajillo wobbles, limberleg	Sympathomimetic amines: *N*-methyl-phenethylamine	Goats Cattle Sheep	6–9 mo or longer	Ataxia, posterior ataxia, proprioception defect of front limbs, fall with forced exercise, weight loss	Recovery likely
Acacia angustissima	Prairie acacia	Unknown: suspected nonprotein amino acids	Sheep		Similar to neurolathyrism: head pressing, twitching, jerking	Used as a protein supplement for sheep
Asclepias sp *A subverticillata* *A fascicularis*	Milkweeds, narrow-leaved varieties contain neurotoxins Horsetail milkweed Mexican milkweed	Unknown; purposed toxin—verticenolide	All animals cattle require twice the dose of sheep	Hours	Depression, muscle twitch, weakness, bloat, salivation, ataxia, seizures. sheep may exhibit a humped-up stance and jackrabbit-like gait	Effects are cumulative dense stands along ditches and hay fields, drying increases palatability, contamination of hay poses significant risk

(continued on next page)

Table 1
(continued)

Plant	Common Name	Toxin; Mechanism of Action	Species Affected	Time from Exposure to Onset of Clinical Signs	Clinical Signs	Notes
Calia secondiflora *Sophora nutrilliana* *Styphnolobium sophora*	Mescal bean, Texas mountain laurel, frijoitol Silky sophora, white loco Affine, Texas sophora	Quinolizidine alkaloids	Cattle acute death occurs Sheep, goats: clinical Signs: usually transient	Hours to days	Cattle: hind leg stiffness, trembling of pelvic and shoulder muscles, unable to rise when they fall. Sheep and goats: signs less severe generally able to walk after short period of time	Leaves and seeds are toxic, *all are suspected to have same toxin and Produce the same clinical signs
Drymaria arenarioides, Drymaria pachyphylla	Alfombrillo, thickweed, inkweed	Saponins	Cattle Sheep Goats	Hours death in <24–48 h possible	Restlessness, diarrhea trembling, dyspnea violent, seizures, coma	Unpalatable, remains toxic when dry, eaten during drought conditions
Karwinskia humboldtiana	Tulidora, coyotillo, buckthorn	Complex anthracenones	Goats Cattle Sheep	Days to weeks	Alertness, increased sensitivity to sound and touch, ataxia, posterior ataxia leading to progressive paralysis	Cumulative
Albizia jilibrissin	Mimosamim mimosa tree	Alkaloids; suspected interference with GABA synthesis	Sheep Cattle Goats	12–24 h	Muscle twitching, trembling, hyperesthesia, salivation, repeat seizures	Rapid ingestion of large quantities of seed pods
Gelsemium semiparvirens	Yellow jessamine, Carolina jessamine	Gelsemine, semipervirine; binds glycine receptors	Cattle Sheep Goats	Minutes	Rapid onset: weakness, convulsive movements of legs	Green in winter

Kallstroemia parviflora	Warty calthrop	Unknown Possible indole alkaloid	Cattle Sheep Goats	Weakness, knuckling of rear fetlocks, walk on carpal joints can continue for months, seizures	Weeks	Occurrence late summer
Zephyranthes atamasca	Carolina lily, swamp lily	Unknown	Cattle	Acute ataxia, collapse, death	Hours	Moist woods and meadows, bulb toxic
Modiola carolina	Carolina Bristle Mallow	Unknown	Goats Sheep Cattle	Ataxia, prostration, seizures, posterior paresis	Weeks	Found in salt marshes and waste areas, requires heavy consumption
Melia azedarach	China berry	Meliatoxins	Cattle Sheep Goats	Salivation, ataxia, trembling, seizures	2–4 h	Drupes and flowers abrupt onset
Peganum harmala	African rue	β-Carbolines, quinolone harman, norharman, tetrahydroharmane	Sheep Cattle Camel	Tremors, ataxia, posterior weakness, narcosis	Days to weeks	Requires large doses unpalatable when green, increases when dry
Astrolepis chohisensis	Jimmy fern, jimmies	Unknown	Sheep Goat Cattle	Violent tremors, arched back, stiff gait, walks backward before seizure, rapid recovery from seizure, can last 2–3 wk	2–3 d	Occurs in winter eliminated in milk, found in limestone hills and mountain slopes
Nicotiana tabacum N glauca	Cultivated tobacco, burley tobacco Indian tobacco	Nicotine; rapidly acting sympathetic and parasympathetic ganglionic depolarizer	Cattle	Excitement, elevation, tremors, weakness, ataxia	Rapid onset	Primarily cultivated tobacco, low risk with wild species

(continued on next page)

Table 1
(continued)

Plant	Common Name	Toxin; Mechanism of Action	Species Affected	Time from Exposure to Onset of Clinical Signs	Clinical Signs	Notes
Eastern United States						
Solidago	Broadleaved goldenrod, hairy goldenrod	Unknown	Sheep	Hours	Rapid onset, muscle tremors of ears and lips progressing to entire body, continual lip and jaw movement, death	Mainly green plant summer and fall but toxin present in hay
Lobelia berlandieri *L inflata*	Berlandier, lobelia Indian tobacco	Pyridine alkaloids: stimulate nicotinic ganglionic receptors	Cattle	Days	Diarrhea salivation drooped ears depression, mydriasis, anorexia, dyspnea, ataxia, coma, death, lingering narcosis	Late winter to early spring
Cephalanthus occidentalis	Buttonbrush	Unknown	Cattle	Days	Rapid onset weakness paralysis seizures	Low palpability, wetlands edges of streams
Laburnum anagyroides	Golden chain tree	Quinolizidine alkaloids; stimulate nicotinic cholinergic receptors	Cattle	Days	Ataxia, salivation, tremors, knuckling of fetlocks	Consumption of leaves

Scientific name	Common name	Toxin	Species	Onset	Clinical signs	Notes
Amianthium muscaetocicum	Staggergrass	Unknown	Cattle Sheep	Hours	Profuse salivation, weakness, ataxia, rapid respiration, dyspnea, anorexia. Greatest risk early spring with green leaves and bulbs	Leaves and bulbs are toxic
Zanthoxylum sp	Prickly ash	Unknown	Goats Sheep Cattle	Weeks	Apparent blindness, high stepping gait, recumbency, struggling, death not common	Moist woods, consumption of bark
Aesculus sp	Ohio buckeye, horse chestnut	Triterpenoid saponnins	Cattle Sheep Goats	1 or more days	Sawhorse stance, trembling, reluctance to move, exaggerated gait, ataxia, seizures possible; generally transient lasting up to 24 h	Leaves, buds, and seeds
Datura stramonium	Jimsonweed, thornapple	Tropane alkaloids: hyoscyamine, scopolamine; anticholinergic: antagonist of acetylcholine at muscuraninic cholinergic receptors	Cattle	Days	Depression, weakness, mydriasis, tachycardia, ataxia	Limited concern: extremely unpalatable when green remains toxic when dry, contamination of hay or feed

(continued on next page)

Table 1
(continued)

Plant	Common Name	Toxin; Mechanism of Action	Species Affected	Time from Exposure to Onset of Clinical Signs	Clinical Signs	Notes
Calycanthus floridus	Carolina allspice, strawberry bush	Indole alkaloids, calycanthine	Cattle Sheep Goats	Rapid onset	Exaggerated reflexes, muscle tremors	Clinical signs similar to strychnine
Cephalanthus occidentalis	California allspice, bubby bush	Unknown	Cattle	Weeks	Hypersensitivity, rigid tetanic seizures with head thrown back	Low palpability, wetlands edges of streams
Ageratina altissmus (Eupatorium rugosum)	White snakeroot	Tremetol; inhibits TCA cycle	Cattle Sheep Goats	Days to weeks	Listlessness, depression, marked weakness, stiffness, tremors	Cumulative effects, excreted in milk "milk sickness"
Western United States						
Halogeton glomeratus	Halogeton, salt clover	Oxalates	Sheep Cattle	Acute onset after 4 h of grazing—death in a few hours common	Sheep: dullness, anorexia, white froth around mouth, hind limb ataxia, seizure with extensor rigidity; cattle: belligerence and progressive stiffness from front to back	Occurs during movement to winter pasture
Corydais caseana	Fitweed	Isoquinoline alkaloids: bicuciine; antagonize GABA	Cattle Sheep	<1 h	Depression, increased respiration and heart rate, disorientation, twitching of face, lips, and ears, ataxia, fall in response to external stimuli seizures	Primarily found in mountain ranges, extremely palatable most often occurs after high spring rainfall or snow

Astragulus *Oxytropis lambertii* *O sericea*	Locoweed, milk vetch Purple loco White loco	Isoquinoline alkaloids: swainsonine bicuciine; antagonize GABA N-oxide	Cattle Sheep	Weeks	Depression; increased respiration and heart rate; disorientation; twitching of face, lips, and ears; ataxia; fall in response to external stimuli seizures	Effects are cumulative, excreted in milk-calf may exhibit illness first, remains toxic in hay
Astragalus miser	Timber milk vetch	Crackerheel nitrotoxin: miserotoxin, 3-nitro-propionic acid, 3-nitro-propano	Cattle Sheep Goats	5 d	Clicking sound (dew claws hit opposite leg) legs when walking, flexion of rear fetlocks, posterior paresis	
Thermopsis rhombifolia	Round leaved thermopsis, mountain pea	Quinolizidine alkaloids	Cattle	Days	Depression, anorexia, arched back, tremors, prolonged recumbency	Dry leaves are toxic
Lupinus sp	Lupines	Quinolizidine, alkaloids; antagonize nicotinic and muscarinic acetylcholine receptors	Sheep* Cattle	24 h	Sheep: muscle twitching, nervousness, head pressing, head butting, seizures Cattle: protrusion of third eyelid, weakness, ataxia, recumbency	*Death in hours to a few days
Aconitum sp	Monkshood, wolfsbane	Diterpene alkaloids: aconitine; blocks closure of sodium channels	Cattle —rare	<1 h	Muscle weakness, dyspnea, must differentiate from larkspur poisoning	High elevation mountain ranges
Isocoma pluriflora	Rayless goldenrod	Tremetol; inhibits TCA cycle	Cattle Sheep Goats	Days to weeks	Listlessness, depression, marked weakness, stiffness, tremors	Cumulative effects, excreted in milk: "milk sickness"

(continued on next page)

Table 1
(continued)

Plant	Common Name	Toxin; Mechanism of Action	Species Affected	Time from Exposure to Onset of Clinical Signs	Clinical Signs	Notes
Achnatherum robustum	Sleepy grass	Probable endophyte producing ergot alkaloids	Cattle Sheep	Hours	Docile, sleepy, lowered head, drag feet when walking lasts up to 24 h in cattle, less in sheep	Toxic green and in hay
Plants that cause stagger syndromes						
Agrostis avenacea	Blown grass	Cornytoxins	Cattle Sheep	Days	Ataxia, rocking stance, high step gait, seizure	Endophyte
Cynodon dactylon	Bermudagrass Bermudagrass staggers	Purposed paspalatrim indole alkaloid	Cattle Goat (mild)	7–10 d	Nervousness, erect ears, tremors, head shaking, ataxia, muscle fasciculation, stiff front legs, seizure, death rare	Mature stands with fungal endophyte Claviceps cynodontis, common and coastal Bermudagrass, fresh and dry
Hilaria sp	Curly mesquite, curly grass, tobosa, big galleta	Claviceps cinera	Cattle Sheep	Days	Tremors, fall when forced to walk recover quickly, seldom fatal	Plant highly resistant to drought and heavy grazing
Lolium perenne	Perennial ryegrass; ryegrass staggers	Lolitrem B and A; inhibit GABA and/or glycine	Cattle Sheep Goats Deer Alpaca	Days	Tremors, stiff, ataxic gait of hind legs, collapse, able to stand and walk after short rest	Produced by the fungal endophyte Neotyphodium lolii, green forage and hay

Paspalum dilatatum *P notatum*	Dallisgrass; dallisgrass staggers Bahiagrass, paspalum staggers	Paspainine, paspalitrems; inhibit GABA and glycine	Cattle Sheep	Hours to days	Nervous, erect ears tremors lips head, neck, and shoulders ataxic gait of hind legs head nodding, hind legs extended and spread apart when standing, collapse, able to stand and walk after short rest	Mature plant, hay
Phalaris sp	Canarygrass	Tryptamine Alkaloids	Sheep Cattle	Acute form: t <24 h on pasture chronic form: weeks	Acute form: excitement nervousness, tremors, stiff hopping gait, collapse, seizures chronic form: recurrent seizures, head nodding, front leg weakness, significant death loss can occur clinical signs of PEM	Not toxic in hay but can occur after several weeks on pasture up to months after removal from pasture, when canarygrass comprises as little as 50% of diet

Data from Refs. [66,68-83]

Postmortem examination seldom reveals any specific gross or microscopic lesions identifying the causative plant; therefore, inspection of the pasture for the presence of toxic plants based on the clinical signs observed and observation that the plants have been eaten is important. Gross and microscopic examination of rumen content for plant fragments aids diagnosis.

With few exceptions, treatment of neurologic disease caused by poisonous plants relies on removal from the offending pasture and symptomatic and supportive care. Many deaths occur due to secondary causes when an animal is left in the pasture, not confined, and not given time to recover.

REFERENCES

1. Cummings BA, Gould DH, Caldwell DR. Identity and interactions of rumen microbes associated with dietary sulfate-induced polioencephalomalacia in cattle. Am J Vet Res 1995;56:1384–9.
2. Cummings BA, Gould DH, Caldwell SR. Ruminal microbial alterations associated with sulfide generation in steers with dietary sulfur-induced polioencephalomalacia. Am J Vet Res 1995;56:1390–4.
3. De Oliverira LA, Jean-Blain DC, Komisarczuk-bony S. Microbial thiamin metabolism in the rumen stimulating fermenter (rusitec); the effect of acidogenic conditions, a high sulfur level and added thamin. Br J Nutr 1997;78:599–613.
4. Amat S, Olkowski AA, Atila M, et al. A review of polioencephalomalacia in ruminants: is the development of malacic lesions associated with excess sulfur independent of thiamine deficiency. HOAJ. 2013. Available at: http://www.hoajonline.com/vetmedanimsci/2054-3425/1/1. Accessed February 10, 2016.
5. Beauchamp RO, Buss JS, Popp JA. A critical review of the literature on hydrogen sulfide toxicity. Crit Rev Toxicol 1984;13:25–56.
6. Kabdykis K. Toxicology of sulfur in ruminants. J Dairy Sci 1983;67:2179–87.
7. Loneragan G, Gould DH, Hamar DW. Association of excess sulfur intake and an increase in hydrogen sulfide concentration in the ruminal gas cap of recently weaned beef calves with polioencephalomalacia. J Am Vet Med Assoc 1998; 213:1599–604.
8. Olkowski AA, Gooneratne SR, Rousseaux CG, et al. Role of thiamine status in sulphur induced polioencephalomalacia in sheep. Res Vet Sci 1992;52:78–85.
9. Sager FL, Hamar DW, Gould DH. Clinical and biochemical alterations in calves with nutritionally induced polioencephalomalacia. Am J Vet Res 1990;51: 1969–73.
10. McAllister MM, Gould DH, Raisbeck MF, et al. Sulphide-induced polioencephalomalacia in lambs. J Comp Pathol 1992;106:267–78.
11. Doughterty RW, Stewart WE, Nold MM. Pulmonary absorption of eructated gas in ruminants. Am J Vet Res 1962;23:205–11.
12. Niles GA. Sulfur induced polioencephalomalacia in weaned beef heifers eating corn gluten feed. 2001. Available at: https://shareok.org/bitstream/handle/11244/11566/Thesis-2000-1 N697s.pdf?sequence=. Accessed March 5, 2016.
13. Olkowski AA. Neurotoxicity and secondary metabolic problems associated with low to moderate levels of exposure to excess dietary sulphur in ruminants: a review. Vet Hum Toxicol 1997;39:359–60.
14. Breves G, Hoeller H, Harmeyer J, et al. Thiamin balance in the gastrointestinal tract of sheep. J Anim Sci 1980;51:1177–81.
15. Rawn JE. The citric acid cycle. In: Biochemistry. Burlington (NC): Neil Patterson Pub; 1989. p. 329–37.

16. Rousseaux CG, Olkowski AA, Chauvet A, et al. Ovine polioencephalomalacia associated with dietary sulphur intake. Zentralbl Veterinarmed A 1991;38:229–39.

17. Amat S, McKinnob JJ, Olkalski AA, et al. Understanding the role of the sulfur-thiamine interaction in the pathogenesis of sulfur-induced polioencephalomalacia beef cattle. Res Vet Sci 2013;95:1081–7.

18. Divers TJ. Neurologic disease, toxic and metabolic encephalopathies. In: Howard JL, Smith RA, editors. Current veterinary medicine 4 food animal practice food. St Louis (MO): WB Saunders Co; 1999. p. 660–1.

19. Jubb KVF, Hustable CR. The nervous system, polioencephalomalacia in ruminants. In: Jubb KVF, Kennedy PC, Palmer N, editors. Pathology of domestic animals. 3rd edition. San Diego (CA): Academic Press; 1983. p. 2179–87.

20. Drewnoski ME, Ensley SM, Beitz DC, et al. Assessment of ruminal hydrogen sulfide or urine thiosulfate as diagnostic tools for sulfur-induced polioencephalomalacia in cattle. J Vet Diagn Invest 2012;24(4):702–9.

21. Drewnoski ME, Pogge DJ, Hansen SL. High-sulfur in beef cattle diets: a review. J Anim Sci 2014;92(9):3763–80. Available at: https://www.animalscience publications.org/publications/jas/pdfs/92/9/3763h. Accessed April 28, 2016.

22. Cebra CK, Cebra ML. Altered mentation caused by polioencephalomalacia, hypernatremia and lead poisoning. Vet Clin North Am Food Anim Pract 2004;20:287–302.

23. Rumbeiha W, Braselton W, Donch D. A retrospective study on the disappearance of blood lead in cattle with accidental lead toxicosis. J Vet Diagn Invest 2001;13:373–8.

24. Bischoff K, Thompson B, Erb H, et al. Declines in blood lead concentrations in clinically affected cattle and unaffected cattle accidently exposed to lead. J Vet Diagn Invest 2012;24(1):182–7.

25. Waldner C, Checkley S, Blakley B, et al. Managing lead exposure and toxicity in cow-calf herds to minimize the potential for food residues. J Vet Diagn Invest 2002;14:481–6.

26. Gwaltney-Brant S. Heavy metals. In: Hascheck WM, Rousseaux CG, Wallig MA, editors. Handbook of toxicologic pathology, vol. 1, 2nd edition. Cambridge (United Kingdom): Academic Press; 2002. p. 701–33.

27. Voigt K, Benavides J, Rafferty A, et al. Lead poisoning in calves associated with eosinophilic meningitis. Vet Rec 2010;167:791–2.

28. Fecteau G, George LW. Lead. In: Anderson DE, Rings SM, editors. Current veterinary therapy food animal practice. 5th edition. St Louis (MO): Saunders; 2009. p. 307–10.

29. George LW. Lead poisoning. In: Smith BP, editor. Large animal internal medicine. 5th edition. St Louis (PO): Mosby; 2015. p. 832–5.

30. Galtney-Brant S. Lead. In: Plumlee KH, editor. Clinical veterinary toxicology. St Louis (PO): Mosby; 2004. p. 204–10.

31. Meldrum JB, Ko KW. Effects of calcium disodium EDTA and meso-2, 3-dimercaptosuccinic acid on tissue concentrations of lead for use in treatment of calves with experimentally induced lead toxicosis. Am J Vet Res 2003;64(6):671–6.

32. Thompson LJ. Lead. In: Gupta RC, editor. Veterinary toxicology: basic and clinical principles. 2nd edition. Boston: Academic Press; 2012. p. 522–6.

33. Morgan SE. Water quality in cattle. Vet Clin North Am Food Anim Pract 2011;27:285–95.

34. Hanna PE, Bellamy JE, Donald A. Postmortem eye fluid analysis in dogs, cats and cattle as an estimate of antemortem serum chemistry values and changes with time and temperature. Can J Vet Res 1990;54:487–94.

35. McLaughlin PS, McLaughlin BG. Chemical analysis of bovine and porcine vitreous humors: correlation of normal values with serum chemical values and changes with time and temperature. Am J Vet Res 1987;48:467–73.

36. Angelos SM, Van Metre DC. Treatment of sodium balance disorder. water intoxication and salt toxicity. Vet Clin North Am Food Anim Pract 1999;15(3):587–607.

37. Angelos SM, Smith BP, George LW, et al. Treatment of hypernatremia in an acidotic neonatal calf. J Am Vet Med Assoc 1999;214(9):1364–7.

38. Abutarbush SM, Petrie L. Treatment of hypernatremia in neonatal calves with diarrhea. Can Vet J 2007;48:184–7.

39. Lieske C, Volmer PA. Nonprotein nitrogen. In: Plumlee KH, editor. Clinical veterinary toxicology. St Louis (MO): Mosby; 2004. p. 130–2.

40. Ortolani EL, Mori CS, Rodrigues Filho JA. Ammonia toxicity from urea in a Brazilian dairy goat herd. Vet Hum Toxicol 2000;42(2):87–9.

41. Meerdink GL. Anticholinesterase inhibitors. In: Plumlee KH, editor. Clinical veterinary toxicology. St Louis (MO): Mosby; 2004. p. 178–80.

42. George LW. Trirayl phosphate poisoning (chronic organophosphate poisoning: dying-back axonopathy. In: Smith BP, editor. Large animal internal medicine. 5th edition. St Louis (MO): Mosby; 2015. p. 999–1000.

43. Pugh DC, Baird AN. Organophosphate polyneuropathy (sheep and goat medicine). Maryland Heights (MO): WB Saunders; 2012. p. 234–6.

44. Lotti M, Moretto A. Organophosphate-induced delayed polyneuropathy. Toxicol Rev 2005;24(10):37–49.

45. Ehrich M, Jortner BS. Organophosphate-induced delayed neuropathy. In: Krieger R, editor. Handbook of pesticide toxicology. San Diego (CA): Academic Press; 2001. p. 987–1011.

46. Mostrum M. Pesticides and rodenticides. In: Smith BP, editor. Large animal internal medicine. 5th edition. St Louis (MO): Mosby; 2015. p. 1611–6.

47. Puschner B. Blue-green algae. In: Smith BP, editor. Large animal internal medicine. 5th edition. St Louis (MO): Mosby; 2015. p. 1595.

48. Roder JD. Blue-green algae. In: Plumlee KH, editor. Clinical veterinary toxicology. St Louis (MO): Mosby; 2004. p. 100–1.

49. VanderKop MA. Strychnine toxicity in livestock. Can Vet J 1993;34:124.

50. Easterwood L, Chaffin MK, Marsh PS, et al. Phosphine intoxication following oral exposure of horses to aluminum phosphide-treated feed. J Am Vet Med Assoc 2010;236(4):446–50.

51. Albretsen JC. Zinc phosphide. In: Plumlee KH, editor. Clinical veterinary toxicology. St Louis (MO): Mosby; 2004. p. 456–8.

52. Osweiler GD. Metaldehyde. In: Osweiler GD, editor. Toxicology. Philadelphia: Lippincott Williams & Wilkens; 1996. p. 250–1.

53. Moeller RB, Puschner B, Walker RL, et al. Determination of the median toxic dose of type C botulinum toxin in lactating dairy cows. J Vet Diagn Invest 2013;15:523–6.

54. Anniballi F, Fiore A, Löfstöm C, et al. Management of animal botulism outbreaks: from clinical suspicion to practical countermeasure to prevent or minimize outbreaks. Biosecur Bioterror 2013;11(Suppl 1):S191–9. Available at: http://online.liebertpub.com/doi/pdf/10.1089/bsp.2012.0084. Accessed April 21, 1016.

55. Payne JH, Hogg RA, Otter HI, et al. Emergence of suspected type botulism in ruminants in England and wales (2001to 2009) associated with broiler litter. Vet Rec 2011;168:640.

56. Johnson AL, Sweeny RW, McAdams SC, et al. Quantitative real-time PCR for detection of the neurotoxin gene of Clostridium botulinum type B in equine and bovine samples. Vet J 2012;194:118–20.

57. Rodloff AC, Krüger M. Chronic clostridium botulinum in farmers. Anaerobe 2012; 18:226–8.

58. Anniballi F, Auricchio B, Delibato E, et al. Multiple real-time pcr sybr green for detection and typing of group III clostridium botulinum. Vet Microbiol 2012;154: 332–8.

59. Fenicia L, Fach P, van Rotter BL. Towards an international standard for detection and typing botulinum neurotoxin-producing clostridia types a, b, e and f in food, feed and environmental samples:a European ring trial study to evaluate a real-time pcr assay. Int J Food Microbiol 2011;145:5152–7.

60. Cunha AC, Moreira GM, Salvarani FM, et al. Vaccination of cattle with recombinant bivalent toxoid against botulism serotypes c and d. Vaccine 2014;32:214–6.

61. Böjnel H, Gessler F. Preence of clostridium botulinum and botulinum toxin in milk and udder tissue of dairy cows with suspected botulism. Vet Rec 2013;172(13): 397–401.

62. Weingart OG, Schreiber T, Mascher C, et al. The case of botulinum in milk: experimental data. Appl Environ Microbiol 2010;76(10):3293–300.

63. Fecteau ME, Sweeny RW. Tetanus. In: Anderson DE, Rings SM, editors. Current veterinary therapy food animal practice. 5th edition. St Louis (MO): Saunders; 2009. p. 283–4.

64. MacKay RJ. Tetanus. In: Smith BP, editor. Large animal internal medicine. 5th edition. St Louis (MO): Mosby; 2015. p. 996–8.

65. Songer JG. Clostridial enterotoxemia (Clostridium perfringens). In: Anderson DE, Rings SM, editors. Current veterinary therapy food animal practice. 5th edition. St Louis (MO): Saunders; 2009. p. 283–99.

66. Borrows George E, Tyrl Ronald J, editors. Toxic plants of North America. 2nd edition. Ames (IA): Wiley-Blackwell; 2013.

67. Michelsen PGE, Smith BP. Clostridium perfringens Type D (enterotoxemia, overeating disease, pulpy kidney disease). In: Smith BP, editor. Large animal internal medicine. 5th edition. St Louis (MO): Mosby; 2015. p. 826–7.

68. Axton Lisa M, Durgan Beverly R. Plants poisonous to livestock. Forage production, University of Minnesota Extension. Available at: http://www.extension.umn.edu/ agriculture/forages/utilization plants-poisonous-to-livestock/. Accessed March 6, 2016.

69. Allison Chris, New Mexico State College of Agriculture, Consumer and Environment Sciences, In: Livestock-poisoning plants of New Mexico rangelands, circular 531. Available at: http://aces.nmsu.edu/pubs/_circulars/CR-531/welcome/ html. Accessed February 25, 2016.

70. John B, Fred Y, Murphy. Plants poisonous to livestock in the southern US. University of Arkansas, North Carolina State University, University of Georgia. Available at: www.uaex.edu/farm-ranch/pest-management/weed/poisonous weed_weed. pdf. Accessed February 25, 2016.

71. Bischoff K, Smith Mary C. Toxic plants of the northeastern United States. Vet Clin North Am Food Anim Pract 2001;27:459–80.

72. Everest John W, Powe Thomas A Jr, Freeman John D. Poisonous plants of the Southeastern Unites States, Alabama Cooperative Extension System Alabama

A&M and Auburn Universities, May, 2005. ANR-975. Available at: http://www.edu/pub/docs/A/anr-0975/an-0975.pdf. Accessed March 5, 2016.

73. F Larry, N Glenn, C Arthur, et al. University of California Agriculture and Natural Resources. Livestock-poisoning plants of California January 2011, publication 8398. Available at: http://anrcatalog.ucanr.edu/pdf8398.pdf. Accessed February 15, 2016.

74. James Lynn F, Panter Kip E, Stegelmeier Bryan L, et al. Astragulus and Oxytropis poison livestock with different toxins, In: Toxicology locoweed research: updates and highlights. 1999. Available at: http://aces.nmsu.edu/pubs/research/livestock range/RR730/toxicology.pdf. Accessed March 8, 2016.

75. Mulligan Gerald A. Plants of Canada and the northern United Sates that are poisonous to livestock, or that have tainted animal products. Available at: http://weedscanada.ca/plants_poisonous_animals.hem. Accessed March 11, 2016.

76. Nice Glenn, Guide to toxic plants in forage. Purdue University Extension WS-37. Available at: http://www.extension.purdue.edu/extmedia/ws/ws_32.toxicplants. Accessed March 6, 2016.

77. Nicholson Steven S. Southeastern plants toxic to ruminants. Vet Clin North America Food Anim 2011;27:447–58.

78. Plants of Texas rangelands. Available at: http://essmeextension/tamu.edu/plants/plant. Accessed March 10, 2011.

79. Plants poisonous to livestock. Department of Animal Sciences-Cornell University. Available at: http://poisonousplants.ansci.cornell.edu/php/plamts.php?action=displayispecies=cattle. Accessed March 5, 2016.

80. Poisonous plant research. Unites States Department of Agriculture Research Services. Available at: http://www.ars.usda.gov/Research/docs.htm?docid=9975. Accessed March 6, 2016.

81. Plants poisonous to livestock in the western states. Unites States Department of Agriculture Research Services; 6011 Agriculture Information Bulletin Number 415. Available at: http://www.ars.usda.gov/is/np/poisonousplants/poisonousplant.pdf. Accessed March 5, 2016.

82. Ralphs Michael H, Stegelmeier Brian L. Locoweed toxicity, ecology, control and management. International Journal of Poisonous Plant Research 2001;1:47–58. Available at: https://www.ars.usda.gov/ARSUserFiles/oc/np/PoisonousPlants/PoisonousPlantResearch.pdf. Accessed March 5, 2016.

83. Stegelmeier Bryan L. Poisonous plants that contaminate hay and forages in the western United States. Proceedings, 2013 Western States Alfalfa and Forage Symposium, Reno NV. Davis (CA): UC cooperative Extension, Plant Sciences Department, University of California; 2013. Available at: http://alflafa.ucdavis.edu/+symposium/proceeding/2013/13was-2_29_stegelmeier_poisonousplants.pdf. Accessed March 5, 2016.

Index

Note: Page numbers of article titles are in **boldface** type.

A

Abiotrophy
    cerebellar
        in ruminants, 61–62
Abscess(es)
    brain
        in calves, 37–39
Aluminum phosphide toxicosis
    in ruminants, 118–119
Anorexia
    in ruminants
        localization of, 23
Ataxia(s)
    cerebellar
        examination of
            in ruminants, 4–5
    proprioceptive
        examination of
            in ruminants, 4–5
    vestibular
        examination of
            in ruminants, 4–5
    without weakness
        in ruminants
            localization of, 21–22

B

Behavior(s)
    change in
        localization of
            in ruminants, 21
Blindness
    localization of
        in ruminants, 20
Body temperature regulation
    difficulty in
        in ruminants
            localization of, 24
Botulism
    in ruminants, 119

Vet Clin Food Anim 33 (2017) 139–151
http://dx.doi.org/10.1016/S0749-0720(16)30092-5
0749-0720/17

Moving?

Make sure your subscription moves with you!

To notify us of your new address, find your **Clinics Account Number** (located on your mailing label above your name), and contact customer service at:

Email: journalscustomerservice-usa@elsevier.com

800-654-2452 (subscribers in the U.S. & Canada)
314-447-8871 (subscribers outside of the U.S. & Canada)

Fax number: 314-447-8029

Elsevier Health Sciences Division
Subscription Customer Service
3251 Riverport Lane
Maryland Heights, MO 63043

*To ensure uninterrupted delivery of your subscription, please notify us at least 4 weeks in advance of move.

Printed and bound by CPI Group (UK) Ltd, Croydon, CR0 4YY

03/10/2024

01040388-0012